AIDS TO PRACTICAL NURSING

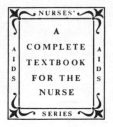

NURSES'

A
COMPLETE
TEXTBOOK
FOR THE
NURSE

AIDS · AIDS

SERIES

THE NURSES' AIDS SERIES

THE GENERAL EDITORS

KATHARINE F. ARMSTRONG
S.R.N., S.C.M., D.N. (London)
formerly Sister Tutor at King's
College Hospital, London, and
Editor of the " Nursing Times "

K. M. BIGGIN
B.A., S.R.N., D.N. (London)
Principal Tutor, The Middlesex
Hospital, London

E. JOAN BOCOCK
S.R.N., S.C.M., D.N. (London)
Principal Tutor at the Royal Free
Hospital, London; formerly Sister
Tutor at St. Thomas's Hospital,
London

MARJORIE HOUGHTON
O.B.E., S.R.N., S.C.M., D.N. (London)
formerly Sister Tutor at University
College Hospital, London, and
Education Officer, General Nurs-
ing Council

WINIFRED L. HUNTLY
S.R.N., S.C.M., D.N. (London)
Principal Tutor at the Royal
Masonic Hospital, London

M. A. NEVELL
B.A., S.R.N.
Sister Tutor at King's College
Hospital, London

MARJORIE WENGER
S.R.N., S.C.M., D.N. (London)
Editor of the " International
Nursing Review "

AIDS TO PRACTICAL NURSING

MARJORIE HOUGHTON
O.B.E., S.R.N., S.C.M., D.N. (London)

Formerly Education Officer, General Nursing Council for England and Wales, and Sister Tutor, University College Hospital, London

and

MARY WHITTOW
S.R.N.

Ward Sister, Medical Unit, University College Hospital, London, and Examiner for the General Nursing Council

with a Foreword by

PROFESSOR M. L. ROSENHEIM
C.B.E., M.A., M.D., F.R.C.P.

Professor of Medicine, University of London. Director, Medical Unit, University College Hospital, London

TENTH EDITION

LONDON
BAILLIÈRE, TINDALL AND COX
7 AND 8 HENRIETTA STREET, W.C.2
1965

First Edition, June 1938
Second Edition, January 1940
Third Edition, October 1941
Fourth Edition, June 1942
  Reprinted, April 1943, *March* 1944,
  December 1944, *February* 1946,
  May 1946
Fifth Edition, February 1947
Sixth Edition, June 1948
  Reprinted, December 1949
Seventh Edition, January 1952
  Reprinted, December 1952, *June* 1954
Eighth Edition, January 1956
  Reprinted, January 1957
  Reprinted, April 1958
  Reprinted, January 1959
  Reprinted, June 1959
Ninth Edition, June 1960
  Reprinted, August 1963
Tenth Edition, January 1965

PRINTED IN GREAT BRITAIN

THE NURSES' AIDS SERIES

THE Nurses' Aids Series is designed to provide a series of text-books in the various fields of knowledge required by the modern nurse. It covers the subjects included in the syllabus of the General parts of the Register and, in addition, includes volumes on certain specialized subjects such as pre- and post-operative nursing, tropical nursing, ear, nose and throat nursing and theatre technique. New volumes are added to the Series from time to time.

Each volume is a complete textbook on its subject (the title "Aids to" indicates that the books are aids to knowledge and not aids to the study of larger books) and is written, except in a few instances, by a Sister Tutor at a prominent hospital. The whole Series aims at providing concisely, clearly and simply just that quantity of information which the nurse needs to possess, gathered together in well-illustrated, easily read and easily carried volumes at a price within the means of any nurse. Judged by the welcome it has received, this aim has been accomplished, and the student nurse has at her disposal a set of convenient, up-to-date, comprehensive textbooks.

THE GENERAL EDITORS

FOREWORD

It is only four years since I was invited to contribute a foreword to the ninth edition of *Aids to Practical Nursing*, and now yet a further edition has been called for. I am not surprised.

The authors bring to the task of producing this book very wide experience, both of nursing and training, and the techniques they describe are those in general use in the United Kingdom. Miss Marjorie Houghton is one of our leading experts on all problems associated with the training of the student nurse, for she was for many years Sister Tutor at University College Hospital before becoming Education Officer to the General Nursing Council. She is joined, in this edition, by Miss Mary Whittow, who is ward sister to one of the Medical Unit wards at University College Hospital, a member of the Council of the Royal College of Nursing and an examiner for the General Nursing Council.

I am always most impressed by the amount of information on all practical aspects of nursing that is to be found in this small volume. The new edition has been extensively revised and once more brought up to date, and I can again most warmly recommend it not only to the nursing profession but also to medical practitioners and students, both as a text book and as an invaluable work of reference.

M. L. ROSENHEIM

University College Hospital,
London.
December 1964

PREFACE

THE NURSES' Aids Series came into existence in June 1938 and *Aids to Practical Nursing* was one of the first three volumes in the Series to be published, the other two covering the subjects of Hygiene and Surgical Nursing. The book has now reached its tenth edition and it is a source of pride and gratitude that it has achieved such wide acceptance in nurse training schools throughout the British Commonwealth during the past twenty-six years.

In preparing this edition we have again tried to bring all the material up to date, omitting procedures which are now generally accepted as obsolete, but giving alternative methods where new ones have not as yet been universally adopted, as for example the supply of "packaged" sterile equipment. The sequence and the content of some of the chapters have been altered, for example "tube feeding" has now been included in a chapter headed "The Use of Intra-gastric Tubes for Feeding, Gastric Aspiration and Lavage". The chapters on "Fluid and Electrolyte Balance" and "Subcutaneous Infusion and Intravenous Therapy" have been re-written, and we are grateful to Dr. C. J. Dickinson of the Medical Unit, University College Hospital, for his help in criticizing and amending this material. The use of the Metric System and the Centigrade thermometric scale is rapidly becoming universal and we have followed the practice now adopted in other volumes of the "Aids" Series of giving the Metric System first followed where appropriate by the Imperial System equivalent in brackets.

Many new illustrations have been introduced into this edition, and for these we have to thank a number of contributors. The Chartered Society of Physiotherapy and the Royal Free Hospital have kindly allowed us to reproduce some of the excellent photographs in their booklet *Lifting Patients in Hospital*. We are most grateful to Miss P. Nuttall, Editor of the *Nursing Times*, for her help in obtaining illustrations, also to Mr. Grima and Mr. Reddick of Oxygenaire Ltd., and to Mr. Cathrall of Down Bros. and

Mayer & Phelps Ltd. for supplying us with illustrations of their firms' products.

Once again Professor Rosenheim has contributed a foreword as he has done for all the previous editions and we would like to thank him for his continuing interest. We should also like to thank Miss E. J. Bocock, Principal Tutor, Royal Free Hospital, for her helpful advice and for reading the manuscript, and the publishers for their never-failing help in the production of this new edition.

MARJORIE HOUGHTON
Kenya.
MARY WHITTOW
London.

December 1964

Acknowledgements for Illustrations

We gratefully acknowledge permission to reproduce illustrations as follows: to Miss S. Treadgold and Baillière, Tindall & Cox Ltd. for Fig. 7.5; to the Chartered Society of Physiotherapy and the Royal Free Hospital for Figs. 7.7–7.14; to *Radiography*, the journal of the Society of Radiographers, for Fig. 9.1; to Photoreportage Ltd. and *Nursing Times* for Fig. 9.2; to the N.E. Metropolitan Hospital Board for Fig. 10.1; to E. & S. Livingstone Ltd. for Figs. 10.2 and 15.7; to Camera Talks Ltd. for Figs. 11.1–11.3, from their 35 mm. filmstrip *Sterilization*, and to *Nursing Times* for Figs. 27.2–3. British Cellophane Ltd. kindly supplied the photograph for Fig. 7.1, and Oxygenaire Ltd. those for Figs. 19.3–4.

CONTENTS

xi

1 THE HISTORICAL BACKGROUND OF NURSING

A study of the historical background of nursing is not only of great interest; it also enables us to understand and appreciate the influence of the past on professional nursing as we know it today. A few of the salient points are briefly outlined in this introduction.

Nursing in Past Ages

Records of the early civilizations show that many of the diseases with which we are familiar are at least as old as history. Ancient India, Egypt, Assyria and Greece gave the physician a place of honour in civil life. Much of the practice of medicine was, however, inextricably mingled with religious practices. In the fourth century B.C. the Greek physician Hippocrates laid the foundation of rational medicine when he stated that disease was due to disordered function of the body, often the result of disobeying the laws of health, and not to the work of evil spirits or the wrath of the gods as was formerly believed. His treatment was based on close clinical observation of symptoms and signs, and his medical notes, clearly but simply written, are still regarded as models.

However, even in Hippocrates' time we find no mention of skilled nursing by specially trained attendants. Treatment was carried out by the physician or his pupil assistants, and the general nursing care of the patient was in the hands of the women of the household or of slaves. Midwives are frequently mentioned in early days, and midwifery was usually a hereditary family profession. The "man midwife" and the obstetric physician were innovations of the seventeenth century.

The Christian Era

The teachings of Christ that service to the very humblest living creature was service to God, and that it was the duty and privilege of the strong to bear the burdens of the weak, inspired the early Christians to seek out those needing help, and to go beyond the narrow limits of their own homes ministering to the bodily and spiritual needs of the sick and poor. The Order of Deaconesses was formed and, working with the Deacons under the Bishops, became the first organized visiting service. A group of wealthy and influential Roman matrons, friends and followers of St. Jerome in the fourth century A.D., also included nursing among their Christian duties, although they did not form an order.

In the mediæval period, when the Church was the great intellectual and social force in all the countries of Christendom, the religious orders were responsible for the care of all who needed help, whether from sickness, poverty or old age. It is interesting to note that many of the large monasteries (some housed 3,000 inmates) had houses both for monks and for nuns, and that the supreme control of the dual establishment was often in the hands of a woman, the Abbess. These women were undoubtedly great figures in their day and age. Their knowledge was wide and their administrative abilities of a very high order.

At the time of the Crusades, in the twelfth century, the military orders were founded. The most powerful and the most famous was the Order of the Knights Hospitallers of St. John of Jerusalem. This order had a "langue" or branch in every country of Christendom. They founded and maintained hospitals first in Jerusalem and later in Rhodes and Malta. The nursing was performed by "serving brothers", but there was a subsidiary women's order whose members nursed in the hospital at Jerusalem, though not in any other hospital of the Order. In the sixteenth century the Order was suppressed in this country, but was re-established in a different form in the nineteenth century. Now everyone is familiar with at least some of its activities, the St. John Ambulance Association and the Voluntary Nursing Corps being the best known.

The Sisters of Charity

In France in the seventeenth century the most important nursing order was that of the Augustinian Sisters. They staffed the largest Paris hospital, the Hôtel-Dieu. These sisters must have been very over-worked. The practice, common at that time, of putting as many as six patients in one bed, made their wards very over-crowded, and in addition to nursing they had to do domestic work, including the washing, which they did in the Seine. Their nursing work was also necessarily limited by the required attention to religious duties, their working day being directed by the priests and not by the physicians. It was not considered suitable that celibate nuns should know much about their patients' bodies or their diseases, so that efficient nursing was hardly possible. The sisters led a life of total self-abnegation and gave loyal and kindly service to the sick, but in those circumstances it was quite impossible that the sick could receive adequate nursing care.

A French priest, Vincent de Paul (afterwards canonized), took an extremely practical interest in the administration of charity both in hospitals and in the homes of the poor, and when visiting the Hôtel-Dieu he was greatly impressed by the need for a more efficient service. With the aid of several influential ladies who had worked with him under the name of "Dames de Charité" in a voluntary visiting service, he took a house in Paris, and there gathered a group of country girls of good character who were to be trained to work in the Hôtel-Dieu with the Augustinian Sisters. His great helper was a Mlle. Le Gras, who became the first Superior of the Sisters of Charity, the nursing community which grew from this small beginning.

St. Vincent instructed the sisters that they were to give implicit obedience to the physicians—this was very revolutionary teaching —and also that they must take no vows nor be tied to a cloistered life, but go wherever they were needed. Indeed, it was not long before the sisters were to be found all over the country, nursing in the homes of the people, in hospitals and in homes for the aged and insane, and from 1654 they rendered service on the battlefield in many campaigns. It is noteworthy that St. Vincent considered that their general as well as their professional education was important, and wished the sisters to have instruction in reading, writing and arithmetic.

The Dark Ages of English Nursing

From the disestablishment of the monastic orders by Henry VIII until the reforms of the nineteenth century, England had no nursing orders comparable with the Augustinian Sisters or the Sisters of Charity. The existing charitable foundations had to staff their institutions with such women as they were able to hire, and the status of nurses was hardly as good as that of a domestic servant in a good-class house. In the private house the patient was nursed by the women of the household or by such "professional nurses" as were available, and there is no doubt that the Dickens' characters Sairey Gamp and Betsey Prig, although caricatures, are representative specimens of that type. The public conscience awakened slowly, stirred by the pioneers and progressive leaders in all branches of science and the professions. The more advanced physicians advocated the training of educated women for real nursing service; the religious bodies, especially the Society of Friends, felt that the appalling social conditions so largely due to ignorance and neglect must be remedied. The latter half of the nineteenth century also saw great advances in medicine, surgery and all scientific knowledge.

Nursing Reforms of the Pre-Nightingale Period

The examples of the communities of the Sisters of Charity in France and the Deaconess Institute at Kaiserswerth near Düsseldorf in Germany inspired the foundation of the many communities in this country in the middle of the nineteenth century. The Kaiserswerth Institute was a new venture that was fast proving itself eminently successful. A German pastor and his wife, Theodore and Frederica Fliedner, had started a small home for discharged women prisoners, and had shortly afterwards added a hospital to their activities. Here they trained a succession of young women of good character and upbringing to be deaconesses. Their duties included nursing in hospital and in the home, home management and the care of young children, and religious visiting. They received practical instruction from the pastor's wife, theoretical instruction in their professional duties from the physicians, and ethical lectures from the pastor. It was an attempt to give an organized training; and though Florence Nightingale, who received practical hospital training at the Institute, clearly saw that the nursing and hygiene could be improved, she was greatly impressed by the moral tone.

Mrs. Elizabeth Fry, of the Society of Friends, knew the Fliedners and their work, and one of her many activities was to found the Protestant Nursing Sisters in 1840. The Park Village Community in north-west London was the first order under the Church of England, but their work was that of visiting rather than nursing. Miss Sellon in Devonport was the head of a band of Sisters of Mercy who gained most of their nursing experience in all too frequent epidemics. Some of these sisters accompanied Miss Nightingale to the Crimea and were often referred to by her as the "Sellonites".

In 1845 St. John's House was started as a training school for nurses under religious direction. The head of the community was a priest of the Anglican Church. The nurses went to King's College Hospital for practical experience and also received instruction from the doctors at the hospital. Later this order took over the entire nursing in that hospital until a lay training school was established in 1885. The St. John Sisters also nursed in the Metropolitan and Charing Cross Hospitals.

The sisters of another Church community, that of All Saints, nursed in the wards of University College Hospital for more than twenty years.

The Nightingale Era

When Miss Nightingale was asked by the Secretary at War, Sidney Herbert, to take a band of nurses out to the Crimea to give the same care to our soldiers that the Sisters of Charity were already giving to the French, the great opportunities of a life of preparation for such a task had come.

This woman of wide education and high social position had from her youth been imbued with the idea that the care and comfort of the sick, and the promotion of health in the family, was work for women of character and education. In spite of home opposition she managed to see all that there was to see of training on the Continent; she was, however, to set standards of practical nursing and hospital administration far in advance of any that she found. At the time of the Crimean War Miss Nightingale was in charge of a small hospital for gentlewomen in Chandos Street.

Her first difficulty when she accepted the task of organizing a nursing service for the army in the Crimea was to find a sufficient number of experienced nurses of reliable character, and to refuse the numerous offers from the totally untrained and unfitted. Florence Nightingale saw that in many quarters this innovation of women in the army hospitals would not meet with favour, and she was most anxious not to take the type of woman who would make the work yet more difficult.

When she arrived in Scutari she found a lack of all provision for the care and comfort of the sick and wounded, and an indifference to this dreadful state of affairs that aroused her to a fury of organization and unsparing work. Conditions were as difficult as they could possibly be, red tape obstructed her on all sides, the army doctors resented the presence of women and, sad to record, her nurses did not all prove suitable, some drank, some were unable to stand the dreadful conditions, others found her a hard supervisor and were continually bickering. Certainly Miss Nightingale spared none, herself least of any.

The soldiers looked upon her as an angel, officialdom regarded her in quite another light, but the public made her their national heroine, and when she returned, broken in health, a grateful country presented her with a large sum of money (£9,000 of which had been subscribed by private soldiers). With this money she founded the Nightingale Training School at St. Thomas's Hospital. The pupils in this school were "trained to train", so that they could in their turn fill important nursing posts throughout the country; and this was only one of the activities of a woman who was almost a continual invalid for the rest of her life, but it was one to which she gave much personal attention.

In addition to laying the firm foundations of the modern system of nursing training, this one woman was responsible for the complete reorganization of civil and military hospitals, and for many reforms improving the sanitation and hygiene of the army, particularly in India.

Professional Organization

The increasing demand for the "Nightingale Nurses" and the opening up of this new profession to educated women meant, of course, that the profession increased rapidly in numbers, and the question of organization and registration on the lines already instituted for the medical profession soon arose. Miss Nightingale herself was opposed to state registration. She always regarded nursing as a vocation, not as a profession, but it is strange that this far-sighted woman could not see the necessity for protecting both the public and the nurses from exploitation by those who were untrained or partly trained.

There is no doubt that the opposition of the most influential person in the nursing world must have been a great factor in delaying state registration for so many years.

The first organized body of trained nurses was that formed by Mrs. Bedford Fenwick in 1887 and known as the British Nurses' Association. Mrs. Bedford Fenwick, before she married Dr. Bedford Fenwick, was Miss Gordon Manson, Matron of St. Bartholomew's Hospital. The B.N.A. was incorporated by Royal Charter and became the Royal British Nurses' Association. With much opposition from within the profession and from without, efforts were made to get a Nurses' Registration Bill through Parliament, but without success. The first Registration Act was passed in 1901, not in England, but in New Zealand.

In 1894 the Matrons' Council of Great Britain and Ireland was formed. In 1898 the council wholeheartedly accepted Mrs. Bedford Fenwick's proposals for an International Council of Nurses. The object was to admit to membership all national nursing groups which had developed, or were trying to develop, professional self-government and a settled professional status. The International Council is mainly concerned with organizing international interchange of nurses, promoting the advance of nursing service and nursing education and the economic and social welfare of nurses throughout the world. It has links with a number of international organizations, including the World Health Organization.

During the long period from 1887 until after the First World War the struggle for registration in England dragged on. In 1916 the College of Nursing was founded by leaders of the nursing profession and by other influential persons impressed with the need for greater professional organization. A draft scheme for the State Registration Act was drawn up. With amendments to this and to the original Bill presented by the Royal British Nurses' Association, a New Bill was sponsored by the Minister of Health, and became in 1919 the Nurses' Registration Act.

The College of Nursing was granted a Royal Charter in 1929; it is now the Royal College of Nursing with headquarters in Cavendish Square, London, and branches throughout England and Wales. A Scottish Board in Edinburgh and a Northern Ireland Committee in Belfast are local headquarters for the Scottish and Northern Ireland Branches. It is the largest organization of Registered Nurses in this country and its activities are many. The professional association department of the College is chiefly concerned with forming and implementing professional policies and giving help where required to the individual nurse. The educational side of the activities of the College covers a wide field in preparing nurses for posts in hospitals and in the fields of public health and occupational health, including preparation for teaching and administration in all these areas.

Until recently the United Kingdom organization in membership with the International Council of Nurses has been the National Council of Nurses of Great Britain and Northern Ireland, which was a federation of professional associations, nurses' leagues and fellowships. In 1962 agreement was reached between the National Council and the Royal College of Nursing that the two bodies should amalgamate to form one united organization which would in future represent British nursing internationally under the name of the " Royal College of Nursing and National Council of Nurses of the United Kingdom". Membership of the new organization is on an individual basis and this national body is therefore no longer a federation of associations and leagues and it should be noted that all registered nurses, whether on the General or a Special Part of the Registers maintained by the Nursing Councils of the United Kingdom, are eligible to apply for membership of the Royal College of Nursing and National Council of Nurses.

The State and Nursing

As has already been stated the first Nurses' Registration Act was placed on the Statute Book in 1919. This Act established the General Nursing Council for England and Wales as the statutory body responsible for forming and maintaining the Register of Nurses. Similar Acts established Nursing Councils with the same functions in Scotland and Ireland. The Council also has the duty of laying down conditions for the approval of hospitals as training schools for nurses, inspection of conduct of hospitals so approved and examinations for admission to the Register. Separate parts of the Register were set up for general trained nurses and for nurses trained in the care of sick children, fever patients and patients suffering from mental illness and mental deficiency. Originally there was a separate part of the Register for general trained male nurses; but subsequently this part was amalgamated with the part of the Register for general trained female nurses.

No further nursing legislation was enacted until 1943, when, under the Nurses Act, 1943, the Council was charged with the duty of forming and maintaining a Roll of Assistant Nurses, inspecting and approving hospitals where such training could be undertaken, and conducting examinations for admission to the Roll. The type of examination which the Council considered appropriate for this type of training is mainly concerned with the candidates' practical nursing ability and is known as the "assessment". Under the 1943 Act the right to use the title of "nurse" was, with a few exceptions approved by the Minister of Health, limited to registered nurses, enrolled assistant nurses and students or pupil nurses undergoing training for admission to the Register or Roll. This Act also gave the Council the responsibility of registering as registered nurse tutors those nurses who are qualified in teaching in schools of nursing.

In 1949 further nursing legislation was enacted, and this Act was designed primarily to "improve the training of nurses for the sick". The main provisions of the Act as it affects nursing training were to give further powers to the General Nursing Council; to enlarge the representation on the Council and to set up in each of the Regional Hospital Areas Area Nurse Training Committees which are concerned with regional matters relating to the training of nurses. One provision implemented, at least partially, a recommendation of both the Athlone and the Horder Committees, namely that finance required for the education and training of nurses should be separated from the expenditure required for the maintenance of the hospital services. In 1957 a further Act consolidated the previous three Nursing Acts of 1919, 1943 and 1949. A private member's Bill, introduced into Parliament by Dame Irene Ward in 1960, had as its main objective the removal of the word "assistant" from the title of the enrolled nurse. This Bill was supported by both parties in the House of Commons and was entered on the Statute Book in March, 1961. It is a measure of the value of the work of the enrolled nurse and the recognition of her place in the nursing profession that this measure had the wholehearted support of the majority of registered nurses.

It should be noted that the duties and responsibilities of the Council are clearly defined and limited by Act of Parliament and by Statutory Rules approved by the Minister of Health.

In 1937 an Inter-Departmental Committee on Nursing Services was set up by the Minister of Health and the President of the Board (now the Ministry) of Education. An interim report was published in 1939 and contained many valuable recommendations for the improvement of recruitment to the profession, and of conditions within the profession, such as the setting up of a Recruitment Centre and the establishment of national scales of salaries for nurses. The outbreak of the Second World War interrupted the work of this committee, but in 1941 the Minister of Health set up a committee under the chairmanship of Lord Rushcliffe to draw up agreed scales of salaries and emoluments for State Registered Nurses employed in England and Wales, and for student nurses in hospitals approved as training schools by the General Nursing Council for England and Wales. The terms of reference were later widened to include nurses in the Public Health field, nurses trained in, or training for, tuberculosis nursing, assistant nurses and nurses employed in mental hospitals. A similar committee was appointed in Scotland. The recommendations of these committees were accepted by the Government and the extra cost involved was borne by the Treasury. The principle of nationally negotiated salaries and conditions of service for nurses in the hospitals and health services is now carried on by the Functional Whitley Council for Nurses and Midwives composed jointly of a Management Side and a Staff Side.

The implementation of the National Health Service Act on July 5th, 1948, brought all hospitals, with a few exceptions, under State ownership. Under this Act every man, woman and child in the country is entitled to medical attention and hospital treatment as and when required. The great majority of the population be-between the ages of 15 and 65 years are either self-employed or working for an employer and therefore pay weekly social insurance contributions. Although only a part of the total sum collected from this source is allocated to the Health Service, medical and nursing treatment is available without charge to the individual. The full cost of the National Health Service represents a very considerable proportion of the total national income, but no one would argue against its importance for the nation and the individual. We have accepted this financial burden as right and necessary both as a means of alleviating suffering and promoting a standard of health which is vital for the future well-being of the nation. It is, however, the duty of all who participate in this work not only to endeavour to foster and maintain high standards of service but also to accept responsibility for ensuring that the nation's money is expended to the best advantage.

Mental Health

The treatment and care of persons suffering from mental illness or mental deficiency was, even at the beginning of the century, largely limited to custodial care which had as its object preventing the patient from harming himself or other people. The admission of patients and the administration of mental institutions were largely dictated by Acts of Parliament, the Lunacy and Mental Treatment Acts of 1890 to 1930 and the Mental Deficiency Acts of 1913 to 1938. Towards the end of the last century the Royal Medico-Psychological Association, a professional association of doctors primarily concerned with and interested in the treatment of mental illness and mental deficiency, initiated a course of training and an examination for men and women working in mental hospitals and mental deficiency hospitals and at that time referred to as "attendants". This step marks the beginning of true professional nursing in these fields. Since then great advances have been made not only in the medical treatment but also in the nursing care of the mentally disordered. As interest in and knowledge of mental illness increased so the old conditions in the asylums, with their padded cells, strait-jackets and locked doors, have given way to the development of the modern conception of the mental hospital as a "therapeutic community". The psychological, physical and social methods used in the treatment of mental patients now makes this a field of service for the nurse where kindness, intelligent understanding, sympathy and an ability to form good personal relationships are of outstanding importance.

The Mental Health Act, 1959, which has been implemented in stages since October, 1959, provides for the treatment of patients suffering from mental disorders on the same basis as that of patients suffering from any type of physical illness. Admission to hospital in the case of mental illness or mental subnormality is now "informal", that is to say the legal requirement that the patient should first be certified as being "of unsound mind" no longer operates, although there is provision for compulsory detention in certain circumstances where this is in the interests of the patient and the public. The Act also places responsibilities on local authorities to provide for the care of the mentally sick and subnormal in the community.

Although special parts of the Register for nurses trained in mental and mental deficiency (now called mental subnormality) nursing were set up when the Register of Nurses was established, the Royal Medico-Psychological Association continued to be a recognized body concerned with the training and examination of nurses in this field. However, in 1947 the Association agreed that they would cease to carry out this function and that the General Nursing Council should be the sole body concerned with the training and examinations for the certificates of mental and mental deficiency nursing. When this change took place it was also agreed that nurses who had trained under the auspices of the Association and held the Association's certificate would be entitled to apply to be registered with the General Nursing Council without undergoing further training or examinations.

2 THE HOSPITAL AND THE COMMUNITY: THE HOSPITAL AND THE PATIENT: THE HOSPITAL AND THE COMMUNITY SERVICES: NURSING ETHICS: HOSPITAL ETIQUETTE

The Hospital and the Community

In the first chapter we tried to indicate in outline how the nursing profession has grown through the ages, sometimes making great strides forward and at other times apparently lost in an age of general indifference to the welfare of the "common man". Just as the progress of nursing has reflected the social outlook of a particular age or century, so also have the hospitals and the health and welfare services.

Student nurses at the time of entry to the training school have to adjust themselves to new surroundings and may be somewhat bewildered by the many aspects of hospital life. The student may also have preconceived ideas about the hospital and about nursing, which bear little resemblance to reality. It may be worth while, therefore, to consider very briefly the function of the hospital in the community at the present time.

First we think of the day-to-day function of caring for the sick who lie in the beds in the wards or enter the casualty or out-patient departments. The hospital has to carry on its work day and night. There can be no moment in the twenty-four hours when the sick are not in need of medical attention and nursing care. This affects not only the medical and nursing staffs but also the ancillary staff and lay workers; porters, orderlies and domestic workers must be available for a twenty-four hour service, and other departments ancillary to medicine, such as dispensaries, laboratories, X-ray and physiotherapy departments, though not always providing a twenty-four hour service, have to cover a long span of hours and often to work at week-ends. These examples will serve to show that the organization of a hospital is, of necessity, complex and makes demands upon its personnel that are not equalled in many other spheres.

We must also consider the educational function of the hospital. In many of our larger hospitals, in addition to the training of nurses, the professional education of doctors, radiographers, physiotherapists, midwives and social workers is carried out. Many hospitals take part in the post-graduate training of medical specialists, although not forming part of an undergraduate medical school. Whatever the part played by the individual hospital in professional education we should not forget the role of the hospitals as health education centres. The aim of treatment is not only to cure or arrest disease but to restore the patient as far as possible to full activity. The co-operation of the patient is needed and he must be informed and instructed so that he can play his part in his own recovery and subsequent welfare.

A third function of the hospital is as an institution for clinical research. Research begins in the laboratory, but discoveries have to be put to the test if they are to have any practical use. In the last century Joseph Lister had theories about safe surgery which would abolish "hospital gangrene" and septicæmia, from which so many patients died in hospital in spite of surgical skill. If, in the face of much opposition and scepticism, he had not had the courage to put his theories into practice "antiseptic surgery" which opened the door to the great surgical advances of the twentieth century, would have been delayed for many years. From the days of Lister's triumphant vindication of his methods, research workers and clinical practitioners have striven to improve on this first great advance in the practice of safe surgery, until in this decade we have seen the discovery of chemical substances which can control sepsis to a degree undreamt of at the beginning of the century. Present-day methods of surgery are a great advance upon the cruder methods of antiseptic surgery, but Lister's work was the starting point. There are many examples which could be quoted to show that the close collaboration between the laboratory worker and the clinical worker in mitigating the sufferings of mankind is truly a part of the hospital service. The nurse is a part of the clinical research team, a team in which habits of accurate recording, observation and meticulous attention to detail are the first essentials.

The Hospital and the Individual Patient

Florence Nightingale once said that the hospital should "do the sick no harm". This somewhat sobering statement is well worth careful consideration. Constant vigilance is needed in all medical and nursing procedures in order that these may be carried out with the highest possible degree of competence. A hospital also needs to lay down and to demand strict observance of regulations designed to protect the patient, as for example in the storage, checking and administration of dangerous drugs, and in the measures necessary to prevent cross-infection in hospital wards. There are also less tangible dangers from which we have to guard the patient to the very utmost of our ability. The separation of a young child from his mother when admitted to a hospital ward, at a time when security and a link with familiar surroundings are most needed, is now recognized as a source of harm to the child which may have lasting effects. It has become the practice of most hospitals to allow the mother to be with her sick child as much as possible and in some instances to help with the care of the child.

Older patients too may have many difficulties in adjusting themselves to the strange and even alarming hospital surroundings and the ward routine. They may be apprehensive about their illness and even more about their dependence on others, particularly the nursing staff, which has been forced upon them by a physical condition. In acute illness most patients will passively accept the necessary return to a childish routine in such matters as being fed, washed and attended to in various ways, but some may resent such attentions very strongly and it is most important to realize this and to explain to the patient not only what the nurse is about to do but the reasons why this particular treatment or attention is necessary. If in addition we consider the burden of anxiety about his family and his work that the patient may be carrying, it is readily realized that mental rest and comfort are at least as important to his recovery as the relief of physical discomfort. Reassurance, explanation and information are all needed, and it is the nursing staff who will supply these to a large extent, remembering that medical details concerning the patient's treatment and the course of his disease will be supplied by the doctor. Confidence in all who look after him during his stay in hospital is a great help towards recovery, and since the nurse is the person who has the most intimate and prolonged contact with the patient the effects of her attitude, her words and her actions have great weight.

Many hospitals issue a booklet of useful information to each patient on his admission, telling him about the hospital and the people who are there to help him and including such items as the times of collection and delivery of letters, the visits of the hospital librarian and the hours of opening of the hospital "shop".

If we remember that the patient is one of a family group from which he has been separated in circumstances of considerable anxiety and stress, we shall realize that his illness and consequent admission to hospital have had distressing effects on normal family life. It is sometimes said that the patient is co-operative, but that the relatives are "difficult". This attitude of the patient's relatives is very understandable; even if the illness is a comparatively trivial one it has disrupted the family and introduced an element of anxiety which is concerned not only with the illness but also with the absence of the father or the mother from the family group. When the patient is visited in the strange surroundings of a hospital ward his relatives may doubt whether these strangers into whose care they have entrusted their invalid are really friendly and sympathetic in their treatment of one sick person amongst so many. To watch an experienced and sympathetic ward sister set about the task of allaying the fears of anxious relatives and establishing their confidence in the hospital and the staff is a most valuable lesson in good human relationships.

The Hospital and the Community Services

Although the nurse training school is based on a hospital or group of hospitals, neither nursing nor medical treatment are, of course, confined within the hospital walls. The three branches of the Health Service, the general medical practitioner, the Local Health Authorities and the hospital must understand each other's role and co-operate in the promotion of health and the treatment of ill-health. The student nurse will have opportunities throughout her training of learning about the care of patients in their own homes, the home nursing and midwifery services, their relationship with the general medical practitioners in the locality, the work of the public health nurse in family health care and her part in preventive medicine, which is largely the responsibility of the Medical Officer of Health and his staff. The student will also hear about the scope and value of medico-social work, probably from the hospital almoner, who can help the patient in many ways while he is in hospital and when he is discharged. It may be that the family is in need of financial help or that the patient will have to change his occupation on account·of his illness, and so contact will be made with his employers or with the Resettlement Officer.

To meet fully the needs of the patient in hospital requires an understanding of his social, economic and family background; restoring the patient to an active life often necessitates the use of the resources of health, social and welfare agencies.

Nursing Ethics

Ethics means a code of moral behaviour, and under the term "Ethics of Nursing" are included the moral qualities and rules of conduct relating especially to nursing. The word "nursing" means nourishing; therefore it has come to mean tending and helping all who need it, especially the sick. The object in training nurses is to provide an adequate service to tend the sick and to help in the preservation and promotion of the health of the community in general.

Those who enter this profession must have a real desire to do the work and must be physically and mentally healthy.

Many qualities of character and mind must be developed or acquired during the period of training. Kindliness, sympathy and a cheerful pleasant manner are essential for the successful management of the sick person and his anxious relations, although the nurse must learn to be firm when necessary for the patient's good.

She is expected to show loyalty and obedience to all those in authority, recognizing that they have had the experience fitting them for such positions. She must show loyalty to her patients by giving ungrudging service and by respecting their confidences and their private affairs, reporting to the sister all matters that might influence the patient's condition, but not discussing these things with others outside the ward.

She should aim to be trustworthy and reliable in all matters, however small. These qualities are essential if the nurse is to develop a sense of responsibility both as an individual and as a member of a team.

She should be ready to accept guidance, and when necessary correction, in the right spirit, using all opportunities to increase her knowledge. No progress is possible without perseverance and self-control. She should cultivate the true professional spirit that shows itself in friendliness without familiarity, and in a readiness to minister to all who need her care without regard to social distinctions, race or creed.

These are the foundations, yet more abilities and qualities must be developed in the course of training and experience; keen, alert powers of observation, the exercise of judgment, discrimination and foresight, swift action in emergencies, accuracy in all statements and records, ability to organize and to work with other people so that all matters affecting the welfare of the sick run smoothly.

Hospital Etiquette

Etiquette is the code of manners or the ceremonial observed in certain circumstances.

It is essential to have certain rules of behaviour laid down in a service where discipline and orderliness are necessary for the welfare and safety of the patients for whom the hospital exists, and where the prompt carrying out of orders by the right person is of prime importance.

The newcomer to hospital life may find such ceremonial strange at first, but she will soon realize that after all it is very little more than the application of ordinary good manners to special circumstances. Physicians and surgeons of the visiting staff are addressed as Doctor, Mr. (or Miss) as appropriate, the resident or "house" staff usually as Mr. or Miss ——; the nursing staff should be given their proper title of Matron, Sister or Nurse. Care should be taken to address patients by their correct names.

Courtesy to visitors is a point of good manners that sometimes gets neglected in the rush of a busy ward, and such a lapse is likely to make a very bad impression. Visitors should always be attended to promptly and pleasantly; if they have to be kept waiting, seats should be provided. Patients' friends should not be admitted without permission unless it is the regular visiting hour.

If a member of the medical staff, the matron or a minister of religion comes to the ward, the sister or senior nurse on duty should be informed immediately.

It is not good manners, and therefore not etiquette, to remain seated when spoken to by one of higher rank, nor to lean against the furniture when so addressed. It is good manners and saves confusion and noise if senior people are allowed to pass first; it is courteous to open doors for them. All these small acts of deference should be done unobtrusively and as a matter of course.

The hospital authorities may decide that certain rules and regulations must be kept in the wards and in the Nurses' Home. A little thought should convince the student nurse that these are designed either for the protection of the patients or the welfare of residents. Rules may at times appear inconsistent with personal convenience, but if we are to establish satisfactory relations in the community in which we live, whether inside a hospital or outside, we have to learn to consider the convenience of others.

3 THE WARD UNIT AND ITS EQUIPMENT; CARE, CLEANING AND MAINTENANCE

During his stay in hospital the ward is the patient's home, it is the place in which, as long as he is confined to bed, he must spend his day, eat and sleep, and where his personal toilet needs must be met. The planning of ward units has received a great deal of attention recently as new hospitals are built and older ones are modernized. Not so very many years ago the majority of patients spent most of their time in hospital in bed and were allowed to be up only for short periods at certain times of the day when convalescent. Now many patients are allowed to get up to go to the bath and to the toilet and often to spend a considerable part of the day out of bed. One feature of the newer ward units is the provision of more washing and toilet facilities and of a sitting-and-dining room where ambulant patients can have their meals, and where such recreations as playing card games and listening to radio and television can be allowed without disturbing ill patients.

The use of colour in decoration and furnishings of hospital wards is another aspect of ward planning on which attention has been focused. Cheerful, pleasing colours for walls and furniture replace the cream, brown and dark green walls and the black iron bedsteads of past years. Flowers have always brought pleasure to sick people, whether at home or in hospital, and now in many wards pictures help to brighten the patients' surroundings.

The reduction of unnecessary noise should be the aim of every hospital and something which the nurse must always have in mind. This depends very much on the effort made by each individual member of the staff, but the provision of equipment which can be handled without noisy clatter (*e.g.* plastic rather than metal bins and pails), is a great help. Moreover in the planning of new buildings the type of construction has a bearing on noise and the provision of central departments for the cleaning and sterilization of equipment and for washing up dishes, should make the ward a much quieter place than it can possibly be when these procedures are carried out in ward preparation rooms and ward kitchens.

The question of cleaning and maintenance has also to be considered in the construction of the ward unit. Ward floors, walls, furnishings and finishings should permit easy cleaning, and the materials used should be able to withstand frequent washing. Cleanliness is not only desirable from the æsthetic point of view, it is the first line of defence in the prevention of cross-infection.

WARD CLEANING AND MAINTENANCE

It is generally accepted that the daily cleaning of the ward and its annexes should be carried out by a domestic staff and not by the nursing staff. There are two very sound reasons for this, one is that nurses need to be free from extraneous, non-nursing duties if they are to have time to give adequate nursing care to all the patients in the ward. The second reason is that dust is liable to be heavily contaminated with pathogenic organisms and therefore there is an increased risk of cross-infection if nurses carry out domestic cleaning duties; the same risk is obviously also present if domestic staff undertake nursing duties.

Nevertheless, it still remains the responsibility of the nursing staff to ensure that the patient's environment is clean, orderly and cheerful and some practical instruction in hygienic methods of cleaning is usually included in the student nurses' preliminary course. Such instruction should emphasize the importance of ward cleanliness for the safety of the patient and the value of the part that the domestic staff play in the ward team.

Rules to be observed in Cleaning

(1) All articles required should be collected before beginning.

(2) Clean dusters, rubbers and clean water should be used.

(3) In order to avoid scattering the dust a damp duster should be used for hospital furniture. Polished surfaces will not be harmed by this treatment if a soft dry cloth is used afterwards to restore the polish.

(4) Method and thoroughness must be practised, otherwise corners and ledges may be omitted and time and energy are wasted in covering the same ground again.

2

(5) All cleaning should be done as quietly and with as little disturbance of the patients as possible. Furniture should be returned to its place as it is dusted, so that the ward presents a tidy appearance.

(6) Care and economy must be practised in the use of cleaning materials. In addition to being wasteful, the too free use of soap, soda and cleaning powders is harmful to painted woodwork, polished surfaces and porcelain glaze. Detergent powders and solutions are harmful also to the skin if used in too strong a concentration.

Walls

Ward and annexe walls must be washable. Glossy paint is most often used for the wards and paint or tiles for the annexes. Periodic wall washing is usually done by male cleaners, and the frequency with which this is done will depend on the type of material and the use of the room; for example, the walls of an operating theatre are washed daily.

Floors

Hardwood, linoleum, rubber and plastics are the materials most commonly used for ward floors. Stone "terrazzo" flooring, tiles or cement, all of which can be scrubbed and mopped frequently are suitable for kitchens, sluice rooms, bathrooms and other annexes.

Ward floors, whatever type of material is used, require periodic washing; most floors are either polished with a "non-slip" polish or given a plastic seal coating, which may or may not be polished. The cleaning and maintenance of ward floors require constant attention as the traffic in and out of the ward and continuous activities make it necessary to remove dust and dirt at least twice a day. The time-honoured method of sweeping the ward morning and evening with a broom has been shown to raise the bacterial content of the air very considerably and obviously dust which has been disturbed, but not removed, will settle again on furniture and floors. Vacuum suction cleaners are in general use in most hospitals, and these are satisfactory, provided that the collecting bag is dust-proof. Alternatively, specially impregnated mops which will gather the dust and prevent scattering may be used on floors which are not suitable for wet-mopping.

Electric Lights

These are dusted daily if they can be reached. Centre lights may be so high that they can be washed only periodically, and this is done by cleaners or by the electricians, who may be responsible for washing all electric light fittings.

When using a wet duster for cleaning electric lights or shades care should be taken to see that switches are first turned off. This precaution should also be taken when bulbs are being removed or replaced.

The best type of shade for large lights is the "hygienic" type, with no flutings or ridges to collect dust.

Metal Fittings

Brass and copper fittings, if not lacquered, are cleaned with metal polish; basin taps, chain and plugs require daily cleaning. Chromium plating and stainless steel have largely replaced brass and copper; these metals are much easier to keep clean as they require washing only with soapy water and finishing with a dry, soft cloth. Brass polish should never be used on chromium-plated articles.

Woodwork

Plain wood surfaces should be scrubbed along the way of the grain with soap and water, well rinsed with cold water and dried as completely as possible.

Painted wood surfaces are washed with soap and water or detergent solution. Abrasive cleaning powders should only be used when it is necessary to remove marks on the paint work as they also remove some of the paint.

Treatment and Preparation Rooms

In most modern hospital wards provision is made for surgical dressings and other sterile procedures to be carried out in a treatment room. Such provision is very desirable from the point of view of safe aseptic practice.

Adjacent to the treatment room there are usually two annexes: one annexe is a "clean" preparation room where instruments and equipment are sterilized, unless these are supplied from a Central Sterile Supply Department, and trolleys are prepared; the other annexe is a "dirty" utility room where used equipment is collected and cleaned and the bin for soiled dressings is kept.

Every possible step should be taken to prevent dust contamination of articles in the treatment and preparation areas, for example by keeping windows closed, reducing traffic as far as possible and providing adequate dust-proof storage cupboards for equipment. Boiling water sterilizers, steel bowls and other steel equipment should be maintained in good condition; in hard water areas daily cleaning with soap and steel wool or other abrasive may be needed. Glass shelves and trolleys should be washed with soap and water or dilute detergent solution. Trolley wheels need periodic cleaning and oiling.

The Ward Kitchen

Gas and electricity should be used with care. Great economy can be effected by immediately turning off when not required, and by not having a fiercer heat than is needed.

The vitreous enamel finish used for gas and electric cookers gives a surface which is easily cleaned, provided that any food or milk spilt on the cooker is wiped away at once.

Saucepans should be cleaned as soon as possible after use. Milk saucepans should be used for milk only, and should be filled with cold water before cleaning. No soda must be used in the cleaning of aluminium ware. Feeding cups require care in washing; the spouts should be cleaned with a bottle brush and then well rinsed.

The nurse is responsible for seeing that all crockery and utensils are perfectly clean when patients' trays are set.

Crockery from infectious cases must be kept separate and washed and boiled after use. In some hospitals all ward crockery is boiled after every meal, and this is the usual practice in tuberculosis and infectious diseases units.

Special feed and milk jugs must be inspected by the nurse before use. All special feeds must be covered and labelled.

Refrigerator cabinets should be washed thoroughly at regular intervals using, when necessary, warm water and soap to remove marks. The addition of baking soda (1 teaspoonful of bicarbonate of soda to 1 quart of water) to the washing water "freshens" the interior of the cabinet and counteracts food odours. Unless the type of refrigerator in use has an automatic defrosting mechanism, regular defrosting is necessary as a thick coating of frost on the freezing unit acts as an insulator and the temperature inside the cabinet will then tend to rise. Defrosting is carried out by turning off the current, or turning the control knob back to a point marked "defrost", removing the ice trays from the freezer unit, and either covering or removing the articles on the shelves. The melting ice collects in the drip tray under the freezer unit. Defrosting can be accelerated by placing a container of hot water inside the freezer unit. When the process is finished and the tray has been emptied and replaced, the interior of the cabinet is dried, the articles are replaced and the control knob is turned to give the required degree of coldness. Any food or liquid spilt on the refrigerator shelves should be wiped up immediately.

Hot dishes should be allowed to cool before being placed in the refrigerator.

Infants' feeds are kept in the refrigerator. Milk is usually delivered in bottles; it should be kept in the coolest part of the larder or in the refrigerator.

Larder shelves must be kept tidy and washed daily. All food must be covered.

Unwanted food, such as surplus vegetables or an unwanted milk pudding, should be returned to the central kitchen, if they are not going to be used that day. For food refuse a "pig pail" is usually provided and the contents are sold for pig food. No tins, tea leaves, paper, egg shells or lemon or orange peel must be placed in this pail. All refuse bins must be kept covered.

When plates are stacked up ready for washing the bits must be removed and all food waste put in the pig pail. A strainer or sink basket will help to prevent the waste pipe of the sink getting blocked with grease and tea leaves.

Any repairs required, such as blocked waste pipes or dripping taps, should be reported at once.

Ward Bathrooms and Sanitary Annexes

Baths and lavatory basins are cleaned with soap and cleaning powder. Special care must be paid to the area under the taps, the overflow and the waste outlet. After use baths may be swabbed with a solution of 2 parts Sudol to 1 part water, left for 5 minutes, then thoroughly rinsed with hot water. Washing bowls and mouth wash mugs should be washed in hot soapy water containing disinfectant, such as Sudol 1 in 40 solution or in a detergent solution, such as Savlon 1 in 40, and rinsed.

Dirty Dressing Pails

It is very desirable that soiled dressing bins and pails should be dealt with in a central station if staff, space and equipment for this can be provided. The containers are collected from the wards by porters, the contents are burnt and the pails are washed, disinfected by steam and returned clean to the wards. If the dressing pails have to be cleaned in the ward annexe they should be washed with a mop and disinfectant (*e.g.* crude phenol type of disinfectant 1 in 10), rinsed with boiling water and turned up to drain. When dry they may be lined with paper. Alternatively, the soiled dressings may be placed in paper containers (using forceps); these containers are then placed in the bins.

Bedpans and Urinals

These are flushed with cold water after use and then cleaned with a mop. Automatic bed-pan washers, in which the bed-pans are enclosed for flushing with hot and cold water, are used in most hospitals. The use of this type of washer has the advantage of keeping the sluice room free from unpleasant odours and also of reducing the handling of bed-pans by the nurses. The automatic bed-pan washer does not sterilize the utensils and, where this is necessary, the best method is by boiling in a large tank sterilizer.

Sputum Containers

Metal sputum mugs are emptied and flushed (the sputum is weighed or measured first if necessary) and then boiled for five minutes. 1 fl. oz. sodium bicarbonate solution 1 in 160 is added before taking the sputum mug to the patient. In some hospitals square tin sputum containers with cardboard linings are used. The inner lining is removed and sawdust added to the sputum, which is then burned. Great care has to be taken when dealing with tuberculous sputum; cardboard containers which are disposed of by burning are generally used. The containers should be collected by a porter specially allocated and instructed in this duty. If the nursing staff have to handle the sputum containers of tuberculous patients, gloves, gown and mask should be worn.

Water Closets

The w.c. pan should be sprinkled with powder containing chlorinated soda and left for half an hour, it is then scrubbed with the lavatory brush and flushed. The brush should be kept in an enamel holder with disinfectant such as Jeyes fluid 1 in 40.

Care of Bedsteads and Bedding

The usual hospital bedstead is made of enamelled iron. At one time black bedsteads were in general use, but in recent years the wards have been brightened by the use of lighter colours and bedsteads are now frequently painted in cream or pastel colours or are given an aluminium finish.

Bedsteads should be dusted with a damp duster. If possible they should be thoroughly washed once a week. The springs should be kept free from dust and rust; for this an oily rag is useful. Any defective springs or broken wires should be reported at once, as the wire frame will sag and the bed is then uncomfortable; also the mattress or bedclothes may get torn.

If a patient is known to have an infection, the mattress may be completely enclosed in a plastic cover which can be discarded when the patient is discharged. If disinfection of the mattress is necessary, horse-hair mattresses, with or without interior springs, are usually disinfected by steam at a pressure of 5 lb. per sq. in. and a temperature of 109°C (228°F) for 30 minutes. Heat disinfection is damaging to rubber mattresses and an alternative method is swabbing with 1 in 20 Lysol or Sudol Solution, followed by thorough washing with soap and water.

Rubber Mackintoshes, Air Rings, Pillows and Air Beds

These articles should be washed thoroughly after use. If disinfection is necessary, they can be soaked for 30 minutes in a 1 in 40 Sudol or Lysol solution, or 1 in 10 Roccal solution. At the end of this period they should be washed with soap and water and dried. They should not be placed on or near hot radiators. Bed mackintoshes should not be folded; they are usually stored on rollers, or may be hung over rollers in a mackintosh cupboard.

Air rings and beds should be tested for leaks before being put away. A little air should be left in to keep the inner surfaces apart. They may be dusted with French chalk.

Rubber articles will perish if oil or greasy substances are allowed to remain in contact with them.

Ward Linen

The Medical Research Council's Memorandum on the control of cross infection in hospitals recommends that great care should be taken in the handling of soiled linen because contamination may occur from discharges and from the scattering of dust particles. The Council also recommends that nurses who are concerned in the care of patients and the conduct of sterile procedures should not sort and count soiled linen.

The Collection of Soiled Linen

A suitable method of collecting soiled linen from the bedside is the use of wheeled trolleys fitted with canvas or plastic bags which can be removed, tied and sent for sorting. Soiled linen should be removed from the ward as expeditiously as possible and sorting should be carried out away from the ward unit. Where the care of incontinent patients involves the frequent changing of heavily soiled linen a special bin should be provided and a "foul washing" machine is usually installed.

There is at present a trend towards centralization of all hospital stores, including linen supplies. In many hospitals the checking of both soiled and clean linen is carried out in a central department. It is very desirable that nurses should handle soiled linen as little as possible in order to avoid contamination of their hands and the possible risk of infecting patients, therefore the central counting of soiled linen has much to recommend it. An added advantage is that the nursing staff is relieved of a task which takes considerable time if checking is to be carried out efficiently. It is also usually claimed that losses of linen are reduced by centralization. Nevertheless the student nurse should understand the proper care of linen and the safeguards necessary to prevent unnecessary damage and loss.

Rules for the Care of Ward Linen

(1) Linen should be used only for the purposes for which it is intended.

(2) Linen should be kept as clean as possible. Frequent laundering of very soiled linen wears out the articles.

(3) All articles should be plainly marked and should be carefully checked before sending to the laundry.

(4) Linen should be carefully checked when received from the laundry.

(5) Linen should be inspected before being put away and any repairs required should be done before it is used.

(6) Lending and borrowing should be avoided if possible in order to reduce the risk of losses.

(7) All badly soiled and stained linen should be dealt with immediately on removal from the bed.

Removal of Stains from Linen

Blood. Soak at once in cold water; when decolorized wash in warm soapy water. If the stain is thick and dried into the material, apply a bleaching agent, either peroxide of hydrogen or ammonia. Rinse well afterwards.

Ink. This should be treated at once by putting the article to soak in cold water or in milk; prolonged soaking, at least twenty-four hours, may be required. Rubbing a paste of salt and lemon juice on the stain and allowing the article to lie in the sun is another method which may be effective. Ball-pen ink stains can be removed by the application of methylated spirit.

Tea, Coffee and Cocoa Stains. Wash in cold water and then pour boiling water on the stain. If not completely removed, apply a bleaching agent and rinse well afterwards.

Fruit Stains. Rub well with salt first and then treat as above.

Rust Marks. Salt and lemon juice and exposure to sunlight may be successful, but these marks are difficult to remove, especially if the linen has been laundered in the meantime.

Iodine. Apply ammonia, rinse and then wash.

Stains Caused by Drugs. Stains from drugs applied to the skin or excreted in the urine are often resistant to removal and may require special methods.

4 PRINCIPLES UNDERLYING NURSING PRACTICE

The statement that nursing is essentially a practical profession is constantly, and rightly, reiterated; the ability to give skilled care to the sick and to assist the physician or surgeon in carrying out the prescribed treatment is certainly one of the main aims of the nurse's training. The thoughtful student may, however, well ask the questions: "What is nursing?" "What are the true functions of the nurse?" "On what principles are these procedures and techniques that are the daily routine of the hospital ward based?" Florence Nightingale in her *Notes on Nursing—What It Is and What It Is Not*, published over one hundred years ago, said that nursing "has been limited to signify little more than the administration of medicines and the application of poultices. It ought to signify the proper use of fresh air, light, warmth, cleanliness, quiet and the proper selection of diet—all at the least expenditure of vital power to the patient." Nursing, in her view, should assist the "reparative processes of Nature".

It is evident that with the great advances in medical and allied sciences the treatment of disease is now vastly more complicated than it was when *Notes on Nursing* was written and that the technical side of nursing, the "medicines and poultices" of a century ago, has accordingly become increasingly emphasized. Nursing, however, is not solely a matter of technical skill, important as this is; the nurse also gives a personal service to each individual, assisting him with, or carrying out for him, those functions which, were he able, he would perform without such help. With these concepts of nursing in mind we can attempt to define some of the major principles of nursing care.

Basic Nursing Care

Basic nursing care is planned to meet the individual needs of each patient for nourishment, physical comfort, cleanliness of person and environment, adequate rest, mental comfort and support, and, where appropriate, occupation and recreation. In some cases, meeting the patient's physical needs is a comparatively simple matter, as for example when the patient is convalescent and can, for the most part, attend to his own wants. He may, however, require considerable help and encouragement in his return to independence and may need the provision of suitable mental and physical activities to aid his return to normal life. In some situations, giving adequate physical care may tax to the full the skill and resources of the nurse; an example of such a case is the severely paralysed patient who may be unable to carry out any bodily functions, including the vital function of breathing, without assistance.

Affording mental comfort and support to the patient entails the establishment of a satisfactory nurse-patient relationship and this is not always an easy matter. The patient may be unable to communicate readily, either because of his condition or possibly because of language difficulties. He may have fears, anxieties or problems which he does not express in words but instead by his attitude, which may be unco-operative or even hostile. If the nurse is to gain the confidence of such a patient she must be tolerant and seek to find the reasons for his behaviour. It is often said that in the busy routine of the ward the nurse has little time to talk to the patient; it is probably more important that she should find time to let the patient talk to her. If the nurse is encouraging and sympathetic the patient will often confide to her his fears, worries, or some information bearing on his illness that he may hesitate to tell to any other person.

The Nurse's Place in the Therapeutic Team

In addition to his need for basic nursing care, each patient will have his special needs in relation to his illness. Many persons may be involved in carrying out the programme of investigations and treatment prescribed by the physician or surgeon who heads the therapeutic team; for example the physiotherapist, the radiographer, the dietitian, the laboratory technician and the medicosocial worker. The nurse, however, is the member of the team who has the most intimate and continuous contact with the patient and it is the nurse who must accurately observe, record and report all necessary data relating to each patient. The reports and charts kept by the nursing staff are essential to the doctor in making a diagnosis and assessing the patient's condition. The value of many of the clinical investigations and laboratory tests which may be ordered depends on the nurse's intelligent understanding of the instructions given for the preparation of the patient and the collection of material. She has the responsibility of carrying out any special procedures assigned to her and of assisting the doctor in his treatment. The surgeon in the operating theatre and in the ward must be able to depend on the nurse's knowledge of the principles of asepsis and on her ability to put these into practice.

Protection of the Patient

Protection of the patient from harm is one of the fundamental principles of nursing care and mention is made in Chapter 2 of some of the hazards to which the patient may be exposed in hospital. Some individuals need special care and protection on account of age, or other condition, which makes them particularly vulnerable (for example: pregnant women, infants, young children and old people). Special hazards must be recognized, and as far as possible avoided, in the nursing of unconscious, paralysed or incontinent patients.

In a wider sense, protection of the individual involves not only the avoidance of unnecessary suffering, but the prevention of illness and the promotion of health. The nurse may play a direct part in this as a public health nurse whose main function is to participate in health education and in such practical aspects of preventive care as immunization programmes. Every nurse, wherever she is working, has, however, a contribution to make to the promotion of health by sound advice and good example in her daily contact with patients and their relatives.

Foresight and Planning

Foreseeing possible dangers or complications is an essential part of nursing. Nevertheless, unforeseen emergencies or accidents can occur inside or outside the hospital and in such circumstances the nurse should be able to act as an informed and responsible person. Foresight with regard to emergencies consists in knowing what to do and how to do it, and this demands frequent review and reappraisal of the most effective action to be taken.

5 GENERAL NURSING CARE

In this chapter and the two following ones some of the aspects of general nursing care are discussed and in describing methods used in carrying out certain procedures the statements are inevitably somewhat dogmatic. The nurse should always remember that modifications in practice often have to be made and the procedure adapted to suit the individual.

Sanitary Rounds

It is the usual practice to give bed-pans or urinals at definite times throughout the day to all patients confined to bed; e.g. the early morning, before the ward is opened after the morning cleaning, and after each meal time. Many patients will, of course, require attention at other than the routine times and this should always be given promptly. The ward is closed to all but the nursing staff during the sanitary round. Privacy for the patient using the bed-pan should always be afforded, and where cubicle curtains are used in the wards this is easily and quickly provided, otherwise screens must be used.

Bed-pans

Bed-pans may be made of enamel ware, porcelain, stainless steel, rubber or thermoplastic material. Stainless steel has largely replaced enamel, which is easily chipped and roughened by frequent boiling, and porcelain, which is heavy and breakable. More recently sanitary utensils made of thermoplastic material, such as polypropylene, have been introduced. This is a tough material, more rigid than some plastics and it will retain its shape when boiled. Other advantages are that it will not chip or break easily and is much quieter in handling than metal utensils. Plastic material is not a good conductor of heat and therefore does not feel cold to the touch. The "Perfection" shape of bed-pan is commonly used, as it fits the contours of the body better than the round shape. A rubber bed-pan may be used for incontinent patients, as it can be left in position without causing as much pressure as the hard rim of the usual type. Urinals are supplied in glass, enamel ware, polythene plastic and stainless steel.

A metal bed-pan should be warmed before giving it to the patient and heated racks are usually provided for this purpose in the sluice annexe. If a heated rack is not available the bed-pan should be warmed under the hot water tap, care being taken to see that it is not more than comfortably warm when given to the patient. Heated bed-pan trolleys may be used, the bed-pans are kept in the racks of the trolley, which is plugged into the electric power point and the heating is thermostatically controlled. The trolley is disconnected and wheeled into the ward for the sanitary round. An unheated trolley may be used for the collection of used bed-pans.

It is usual to cover the bed-pan or urinal when giving or removing it; for this purpose thick paper squares (paper towels) are very suitable as they can be discarded each time after use. Where trolleys are used for both clean and used bed-pans, no cover is usually required.

Toilet

When the bed-pan is brought to the bedside the bedclothes should be turned down leaving the patient covered with a blanket. If an air-ring is used it should be removed before inserting the bed-pan. The patient who is allowed to help himself should be asked to pull his knees up, and the nurse will then assist him by placing her right arm under the lower part of the patient's back and then inserting the bed-pan with her left hand. When the patient has had his bowels open, toilet paper may be insufficient for cleansing purposes and wool swabs, warm water, soap, towel and a receiver for soiled swabs will be needed. Swabs should not be flushed down the sluice sink but should be removed with forceps and placed in the bin provided for the purpose.

Many patients are allowed to get up for washing and toilet purposes and the nurse should know which of these patients require some help. For patients unable to walk the distance to the toilet, wheeled "lavatory chairs" are very useful; the seat of the chair has a space shaped to fit over the water closet pan. A patient who is not able to go to the toilet may find it easier and less of a strain to use a commode at the bedside rather than a bed-pan. One type of commode chair has a shelf below the opening in the seat on which a bed-pan can be placed.

Patients who can attend to their own needs should be given washing water, soap and towel to wash their hands after using the bed-pan. After attending to the sanitary needs of a patient the nurse should wash her hands thoroughly. Hand basins should be provided near all toilets for both staff and patients so that the necessary washing of the hands can be carried out at once.

Bathing

In the Bathroom

When the patient is allowed to go to the bathroom, the nurse should see that all requirements are there, including a dressing gown and slippers, that the windows are shut and the bathroom warm. The bath should be prepared at the correct temperature; about 40·5°C (105°F) is the usual temperature for a hot cleansing bath.

Ward bathroom doors are not as a rule locked on the inside, but a screen may be put round the bath to give the patient a greater feeling of privacy. The nurse is responsible for seeing that the hands, feet and hair receive due attention.

In Bed

Requirements:
A large washing basin.
A supply of hot water.
Soap and two washing flannels.
Two towels.
A nail brush and nail scissors.
Mouth wash, tooth brush and tooth paste.
A brush and comb.
Two bath blankets. If these cannot be kept for the patient's own use, a large bath towel should be provided and the patient's own bed blankets used.

The Bath. The windows on either side of the patient should be closed and the bed screened or the curtains drawn. The hot-water bottle should be refilled and placed at his feet. The top of the bed is then stripped, leaving the patient covered with one blanket. If bath blankets are used, one should be rolled under the patient and the other used to cover him. The gown should be put to warm near the fire or on hot-water pipes.

The water used for washing should be as hot as the nurse's hand can comfortably bear and should be changed when it becomes cool or soiled. The patient's face should be washed first and, if allowed, he will probably like to do this for himself. The neck and ears are then washed and well dried. Each part should be washed quickly and thoroughly, though exposing the patient as little as possible. After the arms have been washed the hands should be well soaped and rinsed in the bowl. The chest and abdomen are washed next, paying special attention to the skin of the umbilicus in dirty or neglected patients. After washing the legs the bowl may be placed on the bed, and the feet well soaped and then rinsed in the bowl.

If the patient is able to help he is given a well-soaped flannel and allowed to wash the groins and between the legs, if not, this must be done for him.

When the patient is turned on his side to have his back washed a second nurse may be required to support him.

When the lower part of the back is being washed special care should be given to the cleanliness of the skin of the anal area and when washing the buttocks the nurse should carefully wash and dry the area between the legs while the patient is lying on his or her side.

When the bath is completed the blankets should be removed, the patient left covered with one of the bed blankets, his gown replaced and the bed re-made.

Necessary attention to the back and other pressure areas is given at the time of bathing and at regular intervals throughout the twenty-four hours. For details of this care see pp. 40–43.

Care of the Mouth

If a patient is able to sit up in bed to clean his own teeth he should be supported in a comfortable position with a towel to protect his jacket and the sheet. He needs a tooth glass or metal mug containing tepid or hot water according to preference, tooth paste, brush and a large receiver or basin. Some patients like to use tooth picks or "dental stimulators" and most will like to finish the process with a pleasantly refreshing mouth wash. If the patient cannot sit up, he should be turned to his left side with the towel spread under his head and neck and the receiver on the towel conveniently placed for him to spit into.

A patient who is not able to assist himself should lie on his side as described above. The teeth are cleaned by brushing systematically with a moist tooth brush and the dentifrice, beginning with the outer surfaces of the front teeth, then with patient opening his mouth widely enough to allow the brush to be inserted between the inner surface of the cheek and the teeth; clean first the teeth on the right side and then on the left side and finally brush the inner surface of the teeth. The patient should be allowed to rinse freely during the process, and if he cannot raise his head sufficiently to use a tooth glass, an angled drinking tube should be provided. The state of the tongue and mouth should be noted during the tooth-cleaning process. False teeth must receive frequent attention, they should be scrubbed in clean warm water with a small brush, using bicarbonate of soda or a special dentifrice. The patient should be given a mouth wash after the dentures have been cleaned and replaced.

In acute illness the mouth requires frequent and careful attention. This is especially important in the case of patients whose fluid intake by mouth has entirely ceased or is limited; regular two-hourly attention should be given. Neglect causes great discomfort and, in the case of a patient able to take little or nothing by mouth, may lead to the serious condition of parotitis (inflammation of the parotid glands). In the case of an unconscious patient the danger of inhaling material into the air passages must always be borne in mind and, in order to prevent this, the foot of the bed should be raised so that the patient's head is at a lower level than his trunk; suction may also be required in these cases.

Where frequent attention to the mouth is needed a tray should be kept at the patient's bedside.

Requirements:

A small bowl containing wool swabs.

Mouth sticks or, if these are not available, a pair of fine clip forceps and a pair of dissecting forceps, in a dish.

Gallipots containing hydrogen peroxide or sodium bicarbonate solution; Glyco-thymoline or other suitable antiseptic; an emollient such as glycerin and borax.

A small receiver for soiled swabs.

A mouth wash such as sodium bicarbonate 1 teaspoonful to 300 ml. (10 fluid ounces) of water, or normal or half normal sodium chloride solution.

The wool swabs are secured on the mouth sticks or the clip forceps and are dipped in the peroxide or bicarbonate solution. Using several swabs all surfaces of the teeth, gums, mouth and tongue are carefully cleaned; the dissecting forceps are used to remove soiled swabs from the clip forceps. This procedure is followed by swabbing with Glyco-thymoline or by a mouth wash. If the patient is able to use a mouth wash the nurse should place a towel and receiver under his chin and support his head.

Hydrogen peroxide, in 2-volume strength, is particularly useful when dried mucus and epithelial debris form crusts (known as sordes); peroxide should always be followed by a mouth wash or swabbing with saline solution to remove the froth that forms. Fruit juices, if allowed, will help to keep the mouth clean and moist by stimulating the flow of saliva and mucus, chewing gum has a similar effect.

Care of the Hair

The hair should be brushed and combed twice a day. Long hair is most comfortably dressed by braiding it in two plaits. Some hospital patients on admission require to have the head combed with a fine-toothed comb and then washed. This is usually ordered at the discretion of the ward sister.

Requirements:
Brush and comb and fine-toothed comb.
Bowl of Dettol or Sudol 1–40, solution.
Receiver.
Wool swabs.

When carrying out this treatment the nurse should stand behind the patient who will then not be able to watch the process.

The mackintosh cape should be placed round the patient's shoulders and the hair first brushed and combed free from tangles. Then dipping the small-toothed comb in the lotion, the nurse should take a small strand of hair and comb it through carefully, afterwards wiping the comb on a swab and inspecting the swab. This is continued until the hair has been carefully combed through.

A head which is found to be infested with lice or their eggs (nits) should be treated at once. Several methods are in use.

Lethane Oil. The infested head is treated by the application of an oil composed of 50 per cent. liquid paraffin and 50 per cent. Lethane 384 Special. Eight partings should be made in the hair, four on each side of the mid-line. The oil is then applied to the scalp from a teaspoon or a dropper and spread by massaging the scalp thoroughly. Following the application the hair should be combed daily to remove dead lice and nits but it should not be washed or brushed vigorously for the following eight days as the aim is to leave the oil on the scalp for sufficient time to kill the parasites. Lethane oil also kills nits.

DDT Emulsion (Suleo). This is applied in the same way as Lethane. The hair may be washed 48 hours after this application.

To Wash the Hair of a Patient in Bed
Requirements:
Two mackintoshes and a mackintosh cape.

A shampoo lotion.

Two towels.

A basin.

A large jug of hot water.

A small jug, such as a pint measure.

A rubber hot-water bottle freshly filled, or a small radiant heat lamp or a hand electric hair drier.

The patient's gown should be slipped down below the armpits and the upper part of the chest covered with a blanket or warm bath towel, and the cape placed round the shoulders over this.

The top of the mattress may be turned under and should be covered with a mackintosh. The second mackintosh should cover the wire spring, and on this the bowl is placed. It is not possible to turn down an interior spring mattress but in this case the patient may be moved down the bed leaving a space at the top of the bed large enough to accommodate the washing bowl; two or three pillows placed under the patient's shoulders will support her while her head rests over the bowl. If the head of the bedstead can be removed the washing bowl can be placed on a chair.

The shampoo lotion should be well rubbed into the scalp, using the tips of the fingers. The hair should then be rinsed by pouring water on from the small jug and the shampooing process repeated. After a second rinsing the bowl is removed and the mattress replaced. The hair should be spread out on a towel with a mackintosh underneath and dried with a warm towel. The use of the hand radiant lamp or an electric hair drier will hasten the drying. If the hair is thick and long it should be combed out gently strand by strand when half dry to prevent it from becoming tangled. If the patient cannot lie down, a bed table may be placed either behind her or in front, as is most convenient, and the bowl put on this.

If a patient's scalp is dry and full of dandruff and the hair cannot be washed frequently, the scalp should be rubbed with a mixture of surgical spirit and water followed by thorough brushing.

Care of the Nails

Finger nails should be kept short and trimmed to the shape of the finger. Toe nails should be cut straight across.

Plenty of soap and a soft nail brush should be used if the nails are dirty, and they should be cleaned after washing while the skin is soft. Olive oil may be applied before washing to loosen in-grained dirt in cases where the patient's hands or feet are very neglected.

Pressure Sores (Bedsores)

Pressure sores are ulcers which are liable to occur in a patient confined to bed especially if his nutritional state is poor. In order to prevent their occurrence the nurse should clearly understand the conditions likely to lead to their formation.

Immediate Causes

Immobility and Pressure. Normally we are constantly changing our position, even when asleep. A very sick person, a patient immobilized in a splint, or a paralysed patient is unable to change his position, and immobility combined with pressure of his body on the bed or against a splint leads to a lack of blood in the area and eventually to tissue necrosis and the formation of an ulcer.

The skin areas most subject to pressure when a patient is lying on his back are the back of the head, the shoulder blades, the elbows, over the vertebral spinous processes in thin patients, the sacral area and the heels. A patient left lying on his side for too long may develop sores over the point of the shoulder, on the hip and over the greater trochanter of the femur.

Friction. The skin will become inflamed and sore from constant rubbing. A very restless patient, such as a child suffering from chorea, may develop sores due to friction unless areas such as heels and elbows are protected by padding.

Moisture. If the skin is constantly wet it becomes sodden, un-healthy and very liable to ulceration. Incontinent patients need constant attention; the use of a silicone barrier cream or aerosol spray to protect the skin is a great help in such cases.

Prevention

Every effort should be made to prevent the occurrence of these ulcers, as they are very slow to heal once they form and also constitute a serious focus for infection and toxæmia. The relief of pressure by changing the patient's position, the encouragement of circulation by massage of the superficial tissues which have been subjected to pressure, and cleanliness of the skin are the most important factors in the prevention of pressure sores. The patient's position should be changed at regular intervals but if his condition makes this impossible, for example a dyspnœic patient in cardiac failure, relief of pressure over the sacral area can be achieved by lifting the patient off the bed for a few moments. A paralysed patient should be lifted and his position changed every two hours so that he is alternately lying on his back, his left side, his right side and in the prone position. In the latter position pillows placed under the legs, just above the ankles, will keep his toes from pres-sing on the bed. Alternatively a short mattress which allows his feet to hang over the end may be used.

In addition to these measures, four-hourly massage of the areas subjected to pressure will assist the circulation in the superficial tissues. It has long been the practice for the nurse to carry out this procedure with the well-soaped palm of her hand, following the massage by rinsing and careful drying of the area. The skin must, of course, always be kept clean and daily or twice daily washing is required, but the too frequent use of soap removes the natural protective oil in the skin and so renders it more liable to damage. Thorough massage with the nurse's dry hand, using a little starch powder to give smoothness, is considered to be a better method.

In cases of prolonged illness additional protein is often needed in the daily diet, because patients whose nutritional intake is deficient in this respect are more liable to develop pressure sores and, should they do so, the ulcers will be very slow to heal.

If the skin shows redness, dark discoloration or bruising, this should be reported immediately and every effort must be made to prevent the skin from breaking.

Various aids can be used to relieve pressure and friction, such as an air ring, or air bed, a sorbo mattress, pads of wool or of sorbo rubber. Pads of wool bandaged on the knees, elbows and heels will prevent friction in restless or emaciated patients. A bed cradle will keep the weight of the clothes from the knees and toes. An alternating pressure pad is useful in providing regular and frequent redistribution of pressure areas, particularly where frequent moving of the patient or changing the position in bed is difficult or inadvisable, as for example in the case of certain injuries or with very heavy patients. The pad, which is made of plastic material, is placed over the mattress and under the bottom sheet. The apparatus consists of a motor operating an air pump and a pneumatic pad containing air tubes. When the apparatus is working alternate sets of air tubes are inflated and deflated.

The bed should be kept free from crumbs and creases. Patched and darned sheets should not be used under the patient. Care should be exercised in inserting and removing the bed-pan in order to avoid any abrasion of the skin; the bed-pan should not be left under the patient longer than is necessary.

The skin should always be carefully dried after washing. Incontinent patients require frequent attention to keep them clean and dry. Whenever the patient is found to be wet or soiled, the parts should be thoroughly washed and then smeared with a mixture of zinc ointment and castor oil, or a silicone barrier cream or aerosol to protect the skin. Damp or soiled bedclothes or gown should be immediately replaced by clean dry ones.

Sores may also occur from the pressure of a splint or plaster. Any complaint of pain or of a burning sensation should be reported at once. If the pressure is not relieved without delay, the part will become insensitive; and although the patient will no longer complain of pain, a large sore may form which will be very difficult to heal.

Treatment

If a pressure sore does occur the treatment will depend upon the size and state of the ulcer. Large sloughing sores may require eusol dressings to aid in the separation of the sloughs, but the particular dressing to be used will be ordered by the doctor. Gentian violet paint, 1 per cent., may be used. Shortwave treatment may be ordered, which will be carried out by the physiotherapist.

Use of Hot-Water Bottles and Other Heating Appliances

Hot-water bottles are commonly used as a means of warming a bed in preparation for the reception of a patient, and some authorities consider that they should be used for this purpose only and should not be left in the bed with the patient. However, a well-protected rubber hot-water bottle can be a source of comfort to a patient, provided that he is fully conscious, able to appreciate heat and to move fairly freely in bed. Even under these conditions the nurse must appreciate that there is still a risk of burning the patient if the cover is insufficiently protected or if it leaks.

In some hospitals it is the practice to fill bottles from the hot-water supply tap, this water will be well below boiling point. Alternatively boiling water is poured into a jug from which the bottle is filled. It should be about two-thirds full, and after expelling the air the stopper is replaced and the bottle inverted and shaken to test for leaking. If this test is satisfactory, the bottle is dried and placed in the cover. The cover should be large enough to enclose the entire bottle including the stoppper, and preferably made of flannel. Some hospitals use two covers on each hot-water bottle.

The danger of placing hot-water bottles in the bed of a patient who is unconscious, paralysed or not able to appreciate sensations of heat or pressure is that the pressure of the bottle against the patient's skin can cause damage, even although the bottle may be properly protected and the temperature of the water it contains may not be hot enough to cause a burn unless associated with pressure.

Electrically heated pads and blankets are very useful for warming a bed ready for the reception of a new patient or a patient returning from the theatre. The blanket should be placed flat in the bed over the bottom sheet and when switched on this should be indicated by a light. There is usually a waterproof covering to protect the interior of the blanket from moisture and in addition the blanket should have a clean cotton cover which can be changed for each patient. Electric blankets should not as a rule be left in an occupied bed and if for any reason this is ordered in a special case, it may be sandwiched between two woollen blankets.

6 ADMISSION AND DISCHARGE OF PATIENTS: LAST OFFICES

Admission of a Patient

When a patient who has been on the list for admission arrives at the ward, he should be given a chair while the necessary forms are completed and the information required is obtained. First impressions are apt to be very lasting; the nurse should remember this and not be brusque or hurried in her manner.

In some hospitals particulars are taken and admission forms completed in a reception room before the patient is taken to the ward.

Information Required. *The particulars generally required from the patient or his relatives are as follows:*

Name and address.

Age.

If married or single, widow or widower.

Occupation—in the case of a child the father's occupation.

Religion.

The address of the nearest relative (if not the same as the patient's address) and the telephone number, or the telephone number of a neighbour or friend willing to take a message.

The name of the physician or surgeon in charge of the case.

The name and address of the patient's general practitioner.

If the patient is a child, it is important to obtain full particulars, including the child's previous medical history, from the parents before they leave the ward. They should also sign a form giving permission for an operation to be performed, or for an anæsthetic to be given if it is at all likely that these procedures will be required.

The relatives should receive a list of articles required by the patient, a list of articles that may be brought in and a permit for visiting at the stated times. If the patient is seriously ill a special

visiting permit is usually given, and the relatives should be told
when to enquire or visit again.

The temperature and the pulse and respiration rates should be
taken and written down.

Unless contra-indicated, either a bath is prepared and the
patient taken to the bathroom, or he is bathed in bed.

The condition of the patient's skin, the presence of any sores,
bruises or scars, and the state of general cleanliness including the
hair, should be reported to the ward sister.

Many patients are allowed to be up for part of the day and
most will therefore require suitable indoor clothing. The provision
of individual wardrobes is very desirable, but if patients' clothes
are stored in a kit-room there should be a shelf and hanging space
for each patient. The clothing of dirty and neglected patients may
be infested with fleas or lice and will need to be disinfected. This
clothing should be placed in a canvas bag and labelled. The usual
methods of disinfection used are steam under pressure or formalin
vapour in an airtight chamber.

Admission of an Emergency Case

When a message is received that such a patient is to be admitted,
the nurse taking the message should, if possible, find out what is
the matter with the patient, so that any special requirements can
be prepared. The bed is prepared as described on p. 57.

Care of Valuables

Any large sums of money in the patients' possession or articles
of value should be reported to the ward sister, so that they may
be locked up. In many hospitals they are taken to a safe and the
patient is given a receipted list.

Any drugs in the patient's possession should be given to the
ward sister, who will keep them for the doctor's inspection.

Discharge of a Patient

When a patient is about to be discharged, the nurse should
ascertain that the patient has ready all the necessary clothing.
Dressings, bandages or splints should be inspected and if necessary, freshly applied immediately before the patient leaves the
hospital. Any instructions regarding future attendance at the

hospital or treatment which is to be carried out at home must be fully and carefully explained to the patient or his relatives. Should there be any criticism of the patient's treatment, or any question about his belongings, the nurse should at once report this to the ward sister, so that the matter can be dealt with before the patient leaves the hospital.

The patient is usually given a discharge form which has to be given to the porter on duty at the hospital entrance.

Practice varies in different hospitals with regard to the routine disinfection of mattresses and pillows by steam or formalin vapour after the discharge of a patient. If such disinfection is not considered necessary, the bedding is removed from the ward, brushed and aired and, if possible, exposed to sunlight. The bedstead and the bedside locker are washed with soap and water or with a detergent solution.

Last Offices

The fact that death has taken place must be certified by the doctor or the ward sister. The relatives should be left alone at the bedside for a few moments. Before leaving the hospital they should be interviewed by the doctor or the sister and also told when to return for the death certificate.

Notification of death is usually sent at once to the Matron's office, the Secretary's office and the Porter's lodge.

Any particular wish on the part of the relatives should receive sympathetic attention. If they have had a long and anxious time at the bedside, or if the death of the patient has been a sudden shock, the nurse should make sure that they are fit to leave the hospital. A quiet room in which to rest for a short time and a cup of tea or coffee should be offered.

When the relatives have left the bedside the top clothes are removed from the bed, leaving one sheet to cover the body, and the bottom sheet, draw sheet and mackintosh under the body.

Air rings, hot-water bottles, cradles and pillows should be removed. The gown should be removed and also any jewellery, unless the relatives have expressed a wish that an article, such as a wedding ring, should remain. Their wishes regarding false teeth should also be ascertained. The eyes should be closed and small pledgets of damp cotton wool may be placed on the lids to keep them closed.

The mouth should be cleaned and then closed. A jaw bandage is often applied, but this may cause discoloration if tight, and a thick pad or small pillow under the jaw may be used instead.

The body should be placed perfectly straight in the bed with the feet together and the arms at the side. One pillow may be left under the head.

The body is then covered with the sheet and left for one hour.

At the end of this time the following articles will be required for completing the last offices:

(1) A gown and clean sheets. These are usually special articles put aside for this purpose.

(2) A washing bowl with warm water, soap, flannel and towels.

(3) Brush and comb; if necessary a small-toothed comb.

(4) Cotton wool.

(5) Dissecting forceps, scissors and sinus or Spencer Wells forceps.

(6) If there is a dressing, a bowl of Sudol or chloroxylenol lotion 1–40, white lint, jaconet and bandages will be required.

(7) Receiver or dirty-dressing bin for soiled swabs and soiled dressings.

(8) A name card on which is written the patient's name, the time of death and the ward, and tape for tying the card to the wrist.

The body should be washed all over, using plenty of soap; the nails should be cleaned and cut short.

The rectum (and in the case of a female patient the vagina also if necessary) is plugged, using cotton wool.

Any dressings are removed, tubes are taken out, a Sudol or chloroxylenol compress is applied and covered with wool and a piece of waterproof material. Bandages should be fastened with a small strip of adhesive tape. Safety pins should not be used for this purpose as a serious infection may result if the nurse pricks her finger.

The hair should be brushed and arranged neatly. A woman's hair, if long, should be plaited and tied with white tape or a ribbon.

The gown should be put on with the opening down the back, the eye pads and jaw bandage are removed.

The name card should then be attached to the wrist and the body wrapped in the mortuary sheet.

The whole procedure should be carried out quietly and the bed should be well screened. It is important that all articles should be collected beforehand, so that the nurses do not need to move the screens at all until the procedure is finished. The body should be taken from the ward as soon as possible.

All bed linen and blankets are sent to the laundry. Bedding is autoclaved, water-proof sheeting, unless "disposable", is soaked in a disinfectant solution such as Sudol 1 in 40 for 30 minutes, then washed, rinsed and dried. The bedstead is washed, using a disinfectant solution if necessary, and dried and the bed is made up with fresh bedding and linen.

All utensils used during the patient's illness and the articles used for the laying out should either be disinfected or boiled. Anything belonging to the patient, no matter how small in value, must be carefully kept. Any important or valuable articles such as jewellery, money, letters or documents, should be made into a separate parcel and given into the charge of the ward sister. Clothes and any articles of food should be made up into two separate parcels clearly marked with the name and bed number and a list of the articles enclosed. These are returned to the relatives who are usually asked to sign a receipt for the articles.

Screens should be left round the bed until it has been freshly made up and everything returned to its normal appearance.

7 BED-MAKING: LIFTING AND MOVING PATIENTS

Bedding

Mattresses and Pillows

Two types of mattress are in general use, the hair-filled mattress and the rubber mattress filled with latex foam. The hair-filled type is firm and hard-wearing and its buoyancy and comfort are increased by the use of interior springs. Latex foam mattresses are firm and comfortable, the surface is non-absorbent and easily washed; with this type of mattress there is no need to use a long waterproof sheet when nursing helpless or incontinent patients.

Both soft and firm pillows are used in hospital wards. Soft feather-filled pillows under the head and shoulders are the most appreciated by the patient, although some people are allergic to feathers. Firm pillows are either hair-filled or made of latex foam. These will not conform to shape of the head, nor can they be shaken up and made to fit into a hollow in the same way as soft feather pillows, but they are useful as a foundation below soft pillows and to give support, for example, under the legs.

Blankets

Blankets woven of soft white wool were until recently universally used in hospital wards as they are light and warm. They have, however, some disadvantages, the most important being that they are damaged by boiling and, even if carefully laundered, tend to become thickened and felted. For this reason woollen blankets are not always changed for clean ones when a patient is discharged, and may, therefore, be responsible for spreading infection. Furthermore, they can add considerably to the dust and fluff in the ward and thereby increase the risk of dust-borne infection. Many hospitals have now replaced woollen blankets with cellular cotton ones which will withstand frequent washing and boiling, these blankets are light and warm, and cotton is less expensive than wool.

Bed Linen

Sheets and pillow cases may be made of linen or cotton, or a mixture of these two materials. Linen has a good appearance and is hard-wearing, but it is more expensive than cotton and some people find linen sheets chilly in cold weather. Draw sheets are made of cotton twill which is more absorbent and a little softer than ordinary cotton sheeting. Draw sheets are usually two yards wide (one yard when doubled) and two and a half yards long, or rather more than twice the width of the mattress, in order to allow the area underneath the patient to be changed by pulling the spare piece across the width of the bed. Counterpanes are usually made of cotton, or a mixture of cotton and any other fabric which is washable. They should preferably be light in weight and light in colour.

Protective Sheeting

Waterproof sheets commonly referred to as "mackintoshes" are used to protect the mattress in the case of a patient confined

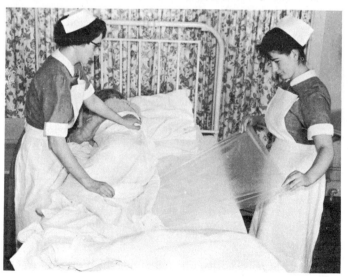

(British Cellophane Ltd.)

Fig. 7.1. A DISPOSABLE WATERPROOF SHEET IN USE.

to bed. For many years rubber has been the most suitable material available for this purpose, a short mackintosh being used to cover the section of the bed under the drawsheet, with an additional long mackintosh covering the entire length of the mattress under the bottom sheet in the case of helpless or incontinent patients. Rubber is however, expensive, is damaged by heat in any form and tends to become hard and uncomfortable with constant use and frequent washing. More recently various types of plastic sheeting have found favour. One such material has a bactericide incorporated in the sheeting and it is also claimed that it will withstand boiling and sterilization in an autoclave. "Disposable" sheeting which is relatively cheap and can be destroyed after use for one patient is also available (Fig. 7.1).

Rubber Rings and Pillows

The square pillow is often more comfortable than the ring, which has a rather hard edge, although the ring is still in common use. A bicycle pump or bellows is needed to inflate air rings, air pillows and air beds. Care should be taken to see that they are not inflated to a degree where they become hard and unyielding instead of soft, as they will then be uncomfortable for the patient. Square pillows of latex rubber may be preferred to air pillows. All rubber rings and pillows should be covered with a cotton case before being placed under the patient.

General Principles of Bed-making

The comfort or discomfort of the sick person largely depends on the bed in which he is lying, its freshness, freedom from creases and crumbs and the proper arrangement of pillows to give support where needed. The prime aim in making the bed is to make the patient comfortable. It is also desirable that the appearance of the bed shall be neat and clean. Disorder and a lack of freshness react unfavourably on the sick person.

All articles required should be collected before beginning to strip the bed. Two nurses should work smoothly together, avoiding unnecessary steps, jarring the bed or jerky movements of the mattress and patient.

The patient must not be exposed during the procedure.

Sufficient help must be available when necessary to move the patient without danger to him and without causing pain.

The actual procedure varies somewhat in different training schools, and it is only possible to indicate the general methods employed for various types of bed.

To Make Up an Unoccupied Bed

Collect the blankets, sheets, pillow cases and mackintosh and place them on a chair at the foot of the bed in the order in which they will be required.

See that the mattress is pulled well up to the bed head. Spread the under blanket over the mattress. Next spread out the bottom sheet, allowing sufficient to tuck in firmly at the foot. Tuck in the sides and the end.

Place the short mackintosh in position across the bed, usually about 18 inches from the head. The draw sheet must be wide enough to cover the mackintosh completely. Tuck in about 1 foot of the draw sheet at one side; at the other side the long end of the draw sheet is pleated or rolled and tucked as smoothly and evenly as possible under the mattress.

Spread out the top sheet, allow about 20 inches at the top, and fold back or tuck in at the foot. Tuck in the sides.

Spread the blankets out, making sure that they will come high enough up to cover the patient's shoulders. Tuck in the blankets at the sides and then the foot; fold the top corners diagonally.

Spread out the counterpane, tuck in the bottom edge, fold the sheet back over the top and finish at the foot end by mitring the corners.

Pile the pillows at the head of the bed with the closed ends of the pillows facing the ward doors.

If the bed is made up ready for the immediate admission of a patient, the top clothes should be left untucked at one side.

To Make an Occupied Bed

It is impossible to give any exact instructions as to which patients may be moved by rolling from side to side and which patients should be lifted, as opinions vary in different hospitals and also change from time to time. As a general rule in surgical cases most patients are allowed and encouraged to move about freely from the first day after operation. In the medical ward patients suffering from congestive heart failure, pneumonia and pleurisy are as a rule nursed sitting up and are lifted for bed-making and sheet-changing.

(1) *If the patient can get up* he should sit at the bedside wrapped in a blanket. The mattress can then be turned and the wire spring dusted as required.

(2) *To make a bed when the patient cannot get out, but may be turned from side to side:*

Place a chair at the foot of the bed.

Strip the counterpane, folding it loosely over the chair.

Strip the blankets separately, folding in the same way, but leaving one covering the patient.

Draw the top sheet down towards the feet, leaving the patient covered with the blanket when the sheet is removed.

Remove all but one of the pillows.

Pull up the mattress if it has slipped away from the head of the bed and dust the bed frame.

Untuck the under clothes, lift the patient's feet, brush out crumbs, straighten the under blanket and sheet.

Find out which side of the bed has the short end of the draw sheet. Roll the patient over towards this side. The nurse on that side of the bed places her hands one under his shoulders and the other under the buttocks and rolls the patient towards her. He must be supported while on his side and a pillow placed under his head.

Straighten the under blanket and sheet on that side, removing any crumbs and tucking the sheet very firmly under the mattress.

Tuck in about one foot of draw sheet and gather the remainder into a roll against the patient's back.

Roll the patient right over on to his other side, supporting him as before. See that he is well covered by the blanket while being turned.

Straighten and tuck in the under blanket and sheet on the opposite side; unroll the draw sheet and tuck it in.

Roll the patient on to his back and then lift him forward with a nurse's hand under each axilla; then one nurse will support him while the other nurse shakes up the pillows and replaces them.

If the patient has slipped down in the bed, lift him up towards the head. See p. 65.

Spread out the top sheet, remove the blanket covering the patient and complete the top of the bed.

(3) *If the patient is sitting upright and may not be rolled from side to side:*

Strip the bed, leaving the patient covered with one blanket. Untuck the sides of the bottom sheet. Lift his legs, brush out the bottom of the bed and straighten the bedclothes. Lift the patient to the foot of the bed, where he is supported by one nurse while the other makes the top part of the bed, shakes up and replaces the pillows.

Lift the patient back and finish the bed as before.

An alternative method that is often practicable, except in cases where the patient is so large that sufficient space is not available, is to lift the patient over to one side of the bed while making the opposite side.

If neither of these methods is suitable then three nurses will be required. When the top bedclothes have been removed, two nurses lift the patient, while the third straightens and tucks in the under blanket, bottom sheet and mackintosh, pulling through the draw sheet.

To Change the Under Sheet

(1) If the patient may be turned on to his side the clean sheet should be rolled or pleated lengthways.

Strip the top of the bed leaving one blanket to cover the patient and turn him to one side. Roll the soiled under sheet with the draw sheet and mackintosh up to the patient's back.

Place the clean sheet in position along the side of the bed, tucking it in and then bringing the roll up to that of the soiled sheet.

Turn the patient over to the opposite side, remove the soiled sheet, spread out the clean one and unroll the mackintosh and draw sheet. Complete the bed in the usual way.

(2) If the patient is not allowed to turn, the sheet should be prepared by rolling it across the width instead of the length, and it is put in from the top instead of from the side.

Untuck the soiled sheet at the head of the bed and roll it down as far as possible.

Tuck in the clean sheet and bring the roll down to that of the soiled sheet.

Raise the patient and remove the draw sheet and mackintosh; pull down the soiled sheet and the clean one.

Raise the patient's legs, removing the soiled sheet and bringing down the clean one.

Lift the patient once more to replace the mackintosh and draw sheet. If the patient is very heavy or helpless, two nurses will be required to lift him while a third removes the draw sheet and pulls down the soiled and the clean under sheets.

In some cases it is permissible to lift the patient down to the foot of the bed after stripping the top clothes. One nurse should support him while the other attends to the top of the bed. He is lifted back when draw sheet and mackintosh have been replaced.

The changing of the bottom sheet may be done from the foot of the bed towards the head. In some instances, *e.g.* a patient with a fracture of the lower limb, this may be the most convenient method.

To Change the Mattress of a Bedridden Patient

The easiest method is to make up another bed as far as the draw sheet and mackintosh, bring it alongside the patient's bed

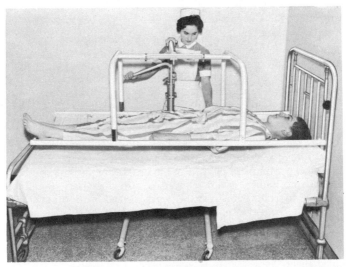

Fig. 7.2. A MECHANICAL PATIENT LIFTER.
The patient being lifted easily from the bed by means of the hydraulic pump.

and then lift him on to the fresh bed. Alternatively a mechanical hoist may be used while the mattress is changed (Fig. 7.2).

Cots

Cots for infants and toddlers are made in much the same way as beds for adult patients, but the counterpane will be tucked in under the mattress at the side instead of hanging down, as is the usual practice in making a bed. The child can usually be removed from the cot and held comfortably by a nurse sitting at the cot side while it is being made. The toddler is likely to spend more of his day sitting on his bed clothes than under them, and therefore in cold weather care must be taken to see that he is sufficiently warmly clad. The cot sides must be pulled up in position and safely fastened before the nurses leave the child.

Special Beds

To prepare a Bed for an Emergency Admission

In most cases the bed is prepared by placing hot-water bottles or an electric blanket in the bed and leaving the top bed clothes untucked at one side so that they can readily be turned back. If a patient is to be received fully clothed, as for example following a street accident, the bottom sheet should be protected by covering it with a long mackintosh and an old blanket or rug, rugs should also be provided to cover the patient.

To prepare a Bed for a Patient returning from the Operating Theatre

General Preparation

The bed is first stripped, the frame dusted with a damp duster and clean linen put on the bottom of the bed. The top bed clothes are made up with clean linen, but are left loose so that they may easily be rolled back when the patient returns from the theatre.

Two hot-water bottles covered with a folded blanket, or an electric blanket, are placed in the bed under the top bedclothes. The pillows are left at the side of the bed.

If the vomit bowl, tongue forceps, gag, swab holder and mops are not on the theatre trolley with the patient, they should be placed ready on the locker at the bedside.

Blocks should be in readiness to raise the foot of the bed.

If hypothermia (lowering of the body temperature) is used in anæsthesia the bed is not heated and the patient is at first covered with a sheet only.

Tonsillectomy

A mackintosh and towel are required to place under the head. Ice and mops must be ready at the bedside. The patient is placed in the semi-prone position on return from the theatre (Fig. 7.3).

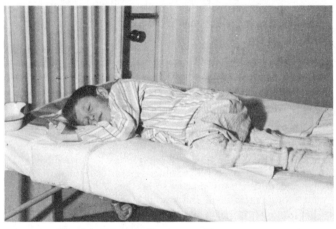

Fig. 7.3. POSITION FOLLOWING TONSILLECTOMY.
Any blood and secretions can easily drain out of the mouth and inhalation is prevented.

Abdominal and Thoracic Operations

The fully upright position with the knee flexed over a pillow was at one time in general use following abdominal operations when the patient had recovered from the anæsthetic and post-operative shock. Now, however, with the encouragement of early movement after operation, it is usual to nurse the patient in a semi-upright position alternating with his lying on his side to assist productive coughing. Recently too, attention has been drawn to the dangers of the upright position even for a patient who has recovered from the immediate effects of the operation

and anæsthetic. Instances have occurred when a patient has
fainted in the upright position and has been prevented from falling
flat by the supporting pillows. If he remains upright his blood
pressure falls rapidly and he may die if not quickly laid flat. Even
if the attack is not fatal there is a possibility that continued low
blood pressure may produce cerebral anoxia with permanent
damage to the brain.

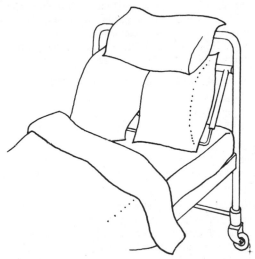

Fig. 7.4. BED PREPARED WITH A BED REST AND THREE PILLOWS
TO SUPPORT A PATIENT IN THE SITTING POSITION.
Two pillows on end are placed against the bed rest and a third
placed across them to support the head and shoulders. The bed
rest and three pillows are a comfortable support and more
economical in pillows and linen than are pillows only. In the
bed illustrated, for a patient with a drainage tube in the thoracic
cavity connected with a water seal bottle, a central gap left
between the pillows prevents kinking or obstruction of the tube.

It may, of course, be necessary in some cases to nurse the
patient in the upright position for purposes of drainage. Such
patients should be kept under close observation, particularly at
night, and should be laid flat at the first complaint or sign of
faintness.

If a patient is to be supported in the upright position as many as six pillows may be needed. The two under pillows may be firm ones, the rest should be feather. The pillows are piled one above the other, supporting the patient's back, and then one soft one is placed well down in the small of the back and a small soft pillow arranged to support the head. Alternatively support may be given by an adjustable bed-rest and three pillows (see Fig. 7.4).

Raising the foot of the bed by blocks or a bed elevator is necessary in order to prevent the patient from slipping down the bed; a support for the patient's feet, such as a large covered sandbag or a padded board and a cradle to take the weight of the bedclothes off the feet will also be required.

Traction applied to a Fracture of the Lower Limbs

The bed is made up with fracture boards under the mattress. An air ring will be required.

The upper part of the bed is made in two sections.

Top. Spread the sheet over the bed, and then a blanket with bottom edge to bottom edge of the sheet. Both together are folded in half, bottom to top and the top edge of sheet is turned out in the usual way.

Bottom. Spread out a blanket with a bottom edge to the edge of the bedstead, turn over at the top where the gap between the sections will be needed. A second sheet may be used under the blanket at the lower half of the bed. Tuck the quilt in at the foot in the usual way and fold over the top edge to correspond with the fold of blanket.

Amputation of Leg

A divided bed similar to that described above may be used for the first forty-eight hours after operation for a patient who has had an amputation of the leg, in order that the dressing on the stump may be easily inspected without disturbing the patient. Many authorities, however, consider this practice unnecessary and undesirable, and the top bedclothes are then tucked in at the foot in the usual manner. A large cradle will be needed, also two sandbags and a cloth or roller towel to steady the stump. In the days when many amputations were undertaken for cases of severe septic infection, a torniquet was usually kept on the bedstead in readiness for any occurrence of secondary hæmorrhage. This type of case is now seldom seen and, moreover, the use of a tourniquet is regarded with disfavour by many surgeons.

Plaster of Paris Splints

Mackintoshes should be put over the bottom sheet under the plaster until it is dry.

A bed cradle is required and the top clothes should be turned back at the bottom to allow free circulation of air.

A blanket next to the patient will keep him from getting chilled.

A large plaster applied to the leg or hip is likely to be very heavy, and the limb may be slung to a Balkan beam when the plaster has set.

Cardiac Failure

In cases of acute carditis which often accompanies acute rheumatism the patient lies flat unless he is short of breath. A patient suffering from congestive heart failure is nursed sitting up, as he can then breathe more easily. If the condition is severe, the patient may not be able to breathe unless sitting upright and leaning forward with his arms supported on a bed table.

Additional requirements are as many pillows as may be necessary; a bed rest, an air ring and a light blanket.

The bed is made up with the draw sheet and mackintosh nearer the head of the bed than usual.

The light blanket is placed next to the patient.

A bed rest helps to support the patient and the pillows are arranged in an armchair fashion.

A bed table, with a soft pillow on it, placed over the bed allows the patient to lean forward for a change of position, and the wide spread of his arms resting on the bed table aids respiration by increasing the capacity of the thoracic cavity.

Patients suffering from congestive cardiac failure are particularly liable to slip down in the bed in spite of all efforts to maintain the necessary support, and the constant moving and lifting required is disturbing to the patient. In addition the patient will make efforts to support himself or to move himself and these will make further demands on an already failing circulation. If possible such a patient should be nursed in a bed which can be adjusted to give a back rest, and raised at the foot end to prevent him from slipping down the bed, and also dropped at the foot end if necessary so that drainage of œdematous fluid can be obtained and the patient given the additional comfort of a "cardiac chair".

Tent Bed

This may be used in conjunction with a steam kettle in respiratory diseases, where it is desired to have a warm moist atmosphere round the patient (Fig. 7.5).

A special frame is attached to the corners of the bedstead and

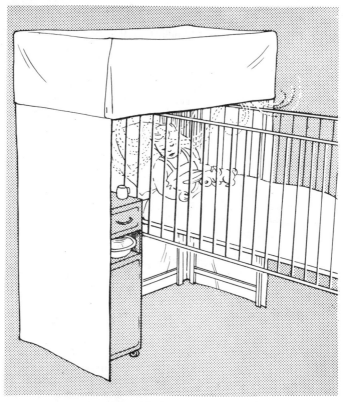

Fig. 7.5. A STEAM TENT.

supports a canopy and the tent sides. The tent may only surround the top half of the bed; if a complete tent is used, then an opening is left at one side. If the special frame is not available, screen frames may be used over which sheets are arranged and pinned.

Prevention of "Foot Drop"

Any patient confined to bed may develop the condition known as "foot drop", but it is more likely to occur in patients who are paralysed and in patients who suffer a long debilitating illness.

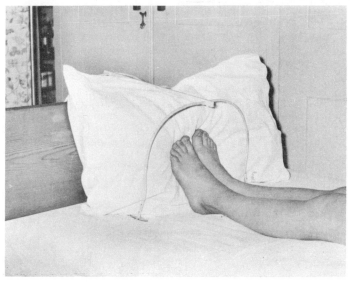

Fig. 7.6. A FOOT SUPPORT IN USE.

The muscles that plantar flex the foot exert more pull than the weaker muscles that dorsiflex the ankle joint, consequently when the patient eventually leaves his bed and should be starting to walk his progress is greatly hampered by foot deformity and by stiffness of the ankle joints. It is part of the nurse's duty to endeavour to prevent the occurrence of foot drop in three ways:

    (i) by supporting the feet at a right angle to the legs by means of a firm pillow padding a board;

(ii) by ensuring that the top bedclothes are never tightly tucked over the patient's feet, a bed-cradle is needed to take the weight of the bedclothes off the feet of a helpless patient;

(iii) by encouraging the patient to move his legs and to dorsiflex the ankle joints at regular intervals throughout the day, or by passively exercising the legs if the patient is unable to move them himself.

LIFTING AND MOVING THE PATIENT

The following pictures which illustrate methods of lifting and moving patients are reproduced by permission of the Chartered Society of Physiotherapists from their publication *Lifting Patients in Hospital*. The two basic methods illustrated are referred to as the "Orthodox Lift" and the "Shoulder Lift", and are used for patients unable to help themselves. Both methods have this in common, since the leg muscles are the strongest in the body—much stronger than the back muscles—it is the leg muscles which are used to lift the patient, the back is always kept straight.

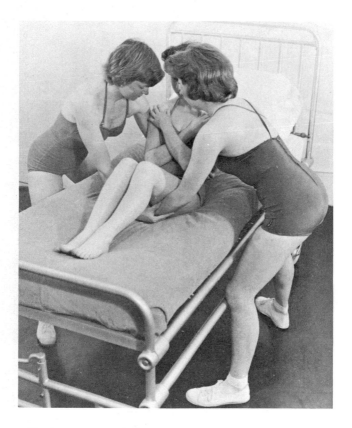

Fig. 7.7. ORTHODOX LIFT. LIFTING THE PATIENT UP THE BED. I.
Note the position of the lifters' hands under the patient's thighs.

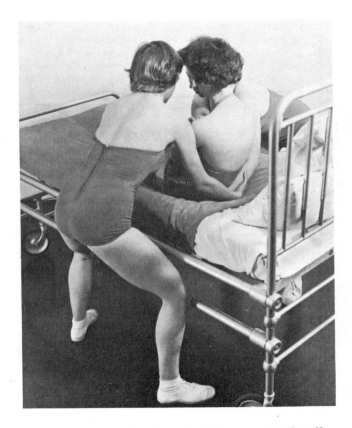

Fig. 7.8. ORTHODOX LIFT. LIFTING THE PATIENT UP THE BED. II.
Note the position of the lifters' feet and legs and the posture of
the head and back. Also note the position of the lifters' hands in
relation to the patient's sacrum. The patient is moved by the
lifters straightening their legs a little and transferring their weight
in the direction of the movement.

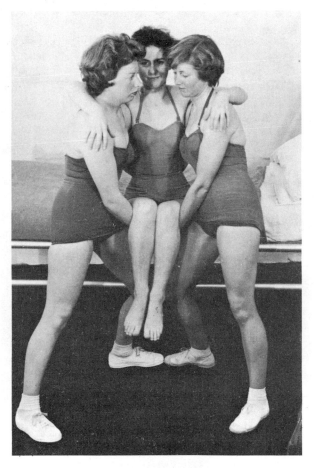

Fig. 7.9. ORTHODOX LIFT. LIFTING THE PATIENT FROM BED TO CHAIR.

Note particularly the bent knees of the lifters, and the positions of their feet. The lifters' hands support the small of the patient's back.

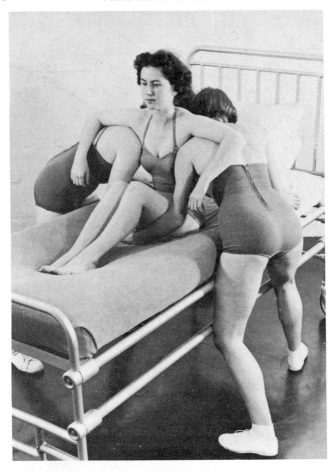

Fig. 7.10. Shoulder Lift. Lifting the Patient up the Bed. I.
Starting position. Note the general position of the lifters in relation
to the patient. It is essential that the lifters stand level with the
patient's hips. One lifter grasps the other's forearm under the
patient's thighs, and each presses her shoulder into the patient's
axilla. The patient should be asked to rest her arms lightly on the
lifters' backs.

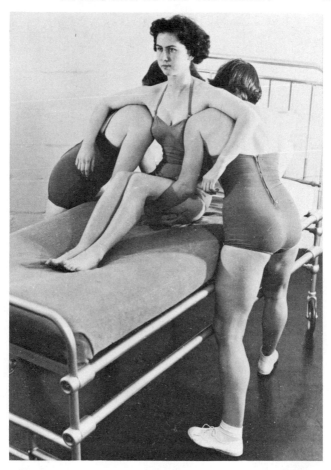

Fig. 7.11. SHOULDER LIFT. LIFTING THE PATIENT UP THE BED. II. The lift. Having pressed her shoulder into the patient's axilla, each lifter smoothly extends her hips and knees and transfers her weight on to the forward leg. Throughout the movement the lifters stand as close to the bed as possible. *Note that* the shoulder lift cannot be used if the patient has injuries to the upper part of the trunk, shoulder or arms.

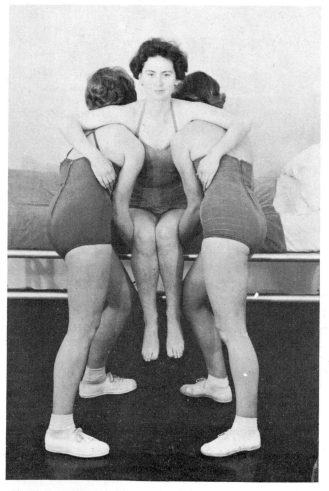

Fig. 7.12. SHOULDER LIFT. LIFTING THE PATIENT FROM BED TO
CHAIR. I.

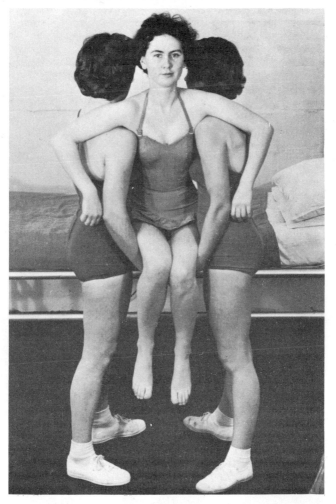

Fig. 7.13. SHOULDER LIFT. LIFTING THE PATIENT FROM BED TO CHAIR. II.

The lift. Having lifted the patient from the bed, each lifter's free hand is placed to support the small of the patient's back. When necessary, one lifter can use this free hand to carry an object, such as a tube or an infusion bottle.

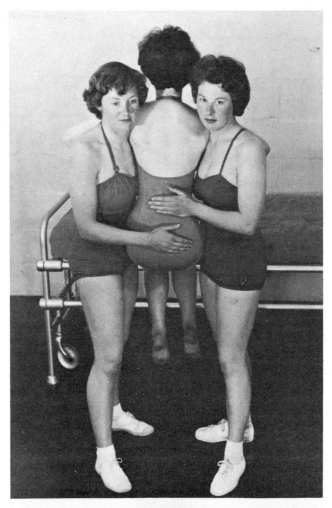

Fig. 7.14. SHOULDER LIFT. LIFTING THE PATIENT FROM BED TO
CHAIR. III.
After lifting, the lifters turn in an agreed direction to face the chair.

8 OBSERVATION AND RECORDING OF TEMPERATURE, RESPIRATION, PULSE AND BLOOD PRESSURE

TEMPERATURE

Temperature is the state of warmth or coldness of a substance or body compared with a standard. The thermometer is the instrument used to register temperature, based on the principle that all matter expands on heating and contracts on cooling. Mercury is a convenient liquid to use for most thermometers because it expands readily with a small change of temperature, quickly assumes the temperature of the body with which it is in contact, and gives a level which is easily read.

Thermometric Scales

Whatever scale is used the fixed points are the same, the boiling point and freezing point of water at normal atmospheric pressure. On the Fahrenheit scale the boiling point of water is marked as 212°F, and the freezing point as 32°F; each degree Fahrenheit is therefore 1/180th of the difference between these two points. On the Centigrade scale the boiling point is marked as 100°C and the freezing point as 0°C; each degree Centigrade is 1/100th of the difference between these two points and 5 Centigrade degrees equal 9 Fahrenheit degrees. The Fahrenheit scale has been generally used in this country, but a change is now being made to the Centigrade scale, which is the internationally recognized one for medical and scientific purposes.

The Clinical Thermometer

This is the type of thermometer used to measure the temperature of the human body. It is a mercury thermometer with a constriction in the tube just above the bulb which causes a break in the mercury thread when the thermometer is removed from contact with the body. The thread of mercury above the constriction therefore remains at the level of the temperature reached until it is shaken down to join the mercury in the bulb.

Most clinical thermometers in use at present are graduated in degrees Fahrenheit, commonly from 95°F to 110°F, although some have a wider range. Each degree is further divided into 0·2°F, thus enabling a patient's temperature to be more precisely recorded. Centigrade scale thermometers for clinical use are becoming available, but it will be some time before they have completely replaced the older Fahrenheit clinical thermometers. The nurse will find, however, that the Centigrade scale is increasingly used in medical notes, textbooks, etc., and therefore she will frequently have to convert a reading from one scale to the other; conversions from Centigrade to Fahrenheit and from Fahrenheit to Centigrade are given on page 124.

Body Temperature

Human beings and all warm-blooded animals keep an almost constant body temperature, the average daily variation being 0·5°C. The normal temperature of the human body is between 35·5°C and 37·2°C, the average being 37°C. Transient rises due to excessive heat production in vigorous exercise or to excessive external heat are soon readjusted.

Heat is produced mainly as a result of muscular and metabolic activity. Heat is lost chiefly through the skin by the evaporation of sweat, by radiation and conduction from the surface of the body, and also through the expired air from the lungs and through the excreta.

The balance of heat production and heat loss is maintained by a heat-regulating centre in the mid-brain, which is sensitive to small changes in the temperature of the circulating blood; a rise in blood temperature results in an increased flow of blood to the surface of the body, increased activity of the sweat glands with increased heat loss by evaporation. At the same time muscle tone is diminished and there is disinclination for further exercise.

A fall in the temperature of the circulating blood produces the opposite effects—constriction of the superficial blood vessels, decreased output from the sweat glands, increased muscle tone with a desire for exercise. The voluntary muscles may show the condition of reflex contraction known as shivering in an endeavour to increase heat production.

Infants and the aged are unable to adjust rapidly to changes in temperature, and are therefore more likely than the normal adult to be readily chilled by exposure to cold and exhausted by excessive heat.

Increase in Body Temperature

A slight daily variation is shown by the normal person, the temperature being highest in the evening as the result of the day's activities, and lowest in the early morning following a night's rest.

In bacterial infections the temperature rises as a result of the increased metabolism; in diseases of the thyroid gland with oversecretion the temperature tends to be higher than normal for the same reason.

Pyrexia is the technical term denoting a raised body temperature.

A rise of temperature above 40°C (104°F) is known as *hyperpyrexia*, and is dangerous to the life of the body cells. Above 43°C (109° to 110°F), life cannot be long maintained. Hyperpyrexia is found in cases of heat stroke, malaria, disorders of the central nervous system and occasionally as a complication after the operation of thyroidectomy. The temperature may be reduced by tepid sponging; evaporation of moisture and cooling of the surface of the body is greatly aided by keeping the air moving with an electric fan.

A rigor is a sudden disturbance of the heat regulating mechanism and commonly ushers in an acute infection, *e.g.* malaria, pneumonia, pyæmic infections. Heat production is in excess of heat loss and the temperature rapidly rises, extreme vasoconstriction makes the surface of the body feel chilly and the patient shivers violently. This stage in a true rigor, as seen in malaria, is followed by a stage of sudden vasodilation, when the patient feels hot and sweats profusely, and as a result the temperature falls.

Continuous Fever. The temperature rises and remains high for a period with very little fluctuation.

In typhoid fever the onset of the fever is gradual, but during the second and third week the chart shows the continuous type of fever. During the fourth week in a favourable case the temperature slowly returns to normal, such a slow defervescence being known as a fall by *lysis*. The course of the fever in this disease will, however, be considerably modified if the infection is cut short by successful chemotherapeutic treatment.

In lobar pneumonia unmodified by chemotherapy the temperature rises abruptly, remains high for about seven days; the fever then terminates by *crisis*.

Remittent Fever. In this type there are marked remissions, the evening temperature being considerably higher than the morning. This is the swinging fever seen in septic infections such as empyema and advanced tuberculosis. Occasionally the "inverse" type will be seen, when the temperature is highest in the morning and lowest in the evening.

Intermittent Fever. In this variety periods of normal temperature intermit with chills and fever. This is characteristic of malaria and may also be seen in pyæmia.

Crisis. This is the term used for a sudden drop from high temperature to normal within a few hours. During this time heat loss is in excess of heat production. The crisis is often accompanied by profuse sweating and polyuria and sometimes by collapse.

Post-operative Variations in Temperature. A careful record of temperature, pulse and respiration, especially in abdominal cases, can be a valuable guide to the patient's condition and may enable the surgeon to recognize a possible complication at the earliest moment. A slight rise of temperature in the first twenty-four hours is usually due to reaction and is not important if the pulse rate and blood pressure are normal. A low temperature with a rapid pulse indicates either a severe degree of shock or hæmorrhage.

A rise of temperature after twenty-four hours, with a slight rise in the pulse rate and a disproportionate rise of the respiratory rate, suggests chest complications. An evening rise of temperature with a corresponding rise of pulse rate from about the third day suggests sepsis.

A slight rise of temperature (about 0·5°C) occurring after the seventh day may be a sign of femoral thrombosis.

Decrease in Body Temperature

At a temperature below 35°C (95°F), the metabolic processes are considerably slowed, and below 30°C (86°F) life cannot be maintained for long.

A lowering of the body temperature may be due to:

(1) Prolonged exposure to cold, especially if accompanied by starvation.

(2) Loss of fluid by hæmorrhage, excessive sweating, vomiting or diarrhœa.

(3) The condition of circulatory depression known as "shock" following severe injuries or operations.

(4) Decreased metabolic rate, *e.g.* myxœdema.

(5) Deliberate cooling of the body to a temperature around 30°C (86°F) or even lower (hypothermia) for a short period in operations on the heart and great blood vessels.

An acute infection accompanied by a subnormal temperature and a rapid feeble pulse is a very grave condition; a sharp rise of temperature with no disproportionate rise in the pulse rate usually indicates a good reaction on the part of the body to the bacterial invasion.

In any illness a sudden fall of temperature without a general improvement in the patient's condition, and without a corresponding fall in pulse rate, is a serious sign.

To Take the Temperature

The clinical thermometer is usually kept in an antiseptic, preferably one of low toxicity, such as chlorhexidine 0·1 per cent. solution, and should be wiped free of this before use. It is very desirable that individual thermometers and containers should be provided for each patient.

The mercury must be shaken down below the lowest mark by a flick of the wrist. The nurse should hold the thermometer well in front of her while doing this, to prevent accidental breakage against the bed or furniture.

The temperature may be taken in the mouth, in the rectum, or in the axilla.

The thermometer must be read immediately after it is removed, and the reading recorded before shaking down the mercury.

Taking the Temperature in the Mouth. The patient is instructed to hold the thermometer under the tongue, closing the lips, but not the teeth.

The temperature must not be taken in the mouth if the patient cannot for any reason close his mouth, if breathing is rapid or difficult, if the mouth is inflamed or sore, or if the patient is irresponsible, *e.g.* an infant, a young child, a delirious, comatose or hysterical patient.

Taking the Temperature in the Axilla. The skin of the axilla must be dried first. The skin surfaces must meet over the thermometer, therefore, this method is not suitable in very thin patients. The thermometer in this position will register 0·25°C ($\frac{1}{2}$°F) lower than in the mouth.

Taking the Temperature in the Rectum. A thermometer of special design with a thick bulb may be used. In any case thermometers used for taking rectal temperature should be kept separate from those used for taking mouth temperatures.

The thermometer should be lubricated and passed 1$\frac{1}{2}$ inches into the rectum; if necessary it should be held in position. The rectal temperature is usually 0·5°C (1°F) higher than the mouth temperature. It gives the most reliable reading, unless the rectum is full of fæces.

Precautions

Thermometers may be marked with the time for which the manufacturers suggest it should be left in position, *e.g.* $\frac{1}{2}$ minute. As a general rule, however, a minimum time of three minutes should be allowed for accurate recording. The patient should be under the nurse's observation during the whole of this time.

RESPIRATION

Respiration is the interchange of gases between the air and the circulating blood in the air sacs of the lungs. The reason for this respiratory act is the constant demand of the living cells for oxygen. The mechanism of respiration depends on the enlargement of the thoracic cavity by contractions of the intercostal muscles and the diaphragm, thereby causing air to enter and expand the lungs (inspiration) and by the recoil of the elastic lungs, forcing air out when the chest wall relaxes (expiration). Although these muscles are voluntary muscles, normal breathing is an automatic action, controlled by a centre in the medulla of the brain sensitive to the amount of carbonic acid in the blood. It is not possible to hold the breath for more than a limited time. A rise of the blood carbonic acid stimulates the centre to send urgent messages to the respiratory muscles, resulting in their contraction. Inhalation of carbonic acid gas (carbon dioxide) has the same effect, and may be used to stimulate respiration.

The pressure in the lungs equals atmospheric pressure, but varies a little with inspiration and expiration. The pressure in the pleural space is always negative and if, by accident or design, air is introduced into this space, equalizing the pressure there with that of the atmosphere, the lung will collapse.

All types of physical exertion increase oxygen consumption, therefore if a patient is suffering from any condition which reduces the oxygen supply to the tissues, for example cardiac failure, complete bed rest forms an important part of his nursing care.

Taking the Respiratory Rate

The normal adult respiratory rate is between 15 and 20 per minute, but this will be increased during exercise or as a result of emotion. In infancy and childhood respiration is quicker than in the adult, being 35 to 40 in a new-born infant and about 25 per minute in a child of five years. The rate should be counted without the patient's knowledge, as control of the chest movements may be voluntary for a period. The usual method is to observe the rise and fall of the chest while still keeping the fingers on the pulse. The number of respirations may be counted for half a minute and doubled, but if there is any irregularity the count should be made for the full minute. The regularity, depth and character of the respirations should be noted at the same time.

Terms Used to Describe Particular Types of Respiration

(1) *Sighing Respiration.* This is known as air hunger. Long deep inspirations, indicating a need for more oxygen, occur in cases of severe hæmorrhage and may also be seen in diabetic coma and in uræmia; it is then described as "acidotic" breathing.

(2) *Slow Respiration.* This is present in coma due to cerebral causes or to large doses of sedative drugs. Excessively slow breathing is a characteristic of poisoning by opium or one of its derivatives.

(3) *Shallow Breathing.* This type of breathing is seen in diseases of the lung, such as pneumonia, and in conditions where the respiratory movements are painful, for example, fractured ribs or pleurisy. Shallow breathing, which is at the same time slow, is seen in cerebral depression.

A tendency to shallow breathing is common in patients who have undergone an upper abdominal operation such as cholecystectomy or gastrectomy and deep breathing exercises are usually given in these cases.

(4) *Stertorous Breathing.* Noisy, snoring inspirations occur in deeply unconscious patients and may be due to the tongue slipping back and blocking the airway. A peculiar hissing respiration may be noted in patients in uræmic coma.

(5) *Stridor.* Stridor, or noisy inspiration, occurs in obstruction of the upper air passages. The noise may be harsh and grating, or may be a whistling sound.

(6) *Wheezing.* This is the term which describes the sounds made during expiration when there is obstruction in the lower air passages, *e.g.* in cases of asthma.

(7) *Apnœa.* This term is used to denote cessation of respiration for a period.

(8) *Hyperpnœa.* This means forced breathing in which the respirations are deep and rapid.

(9) *Dyspnœa.* Breathing is laboured and difficult. The difficulty may be in inspiration, as in laryngeal obstruction, or in expiration, as in asthma.

(10) *Orthopnœa.* This term describes the condition in which the patient is unable to breathe easily unless he is sitting in an upright position; it is frequently seen in cases of congestive cardiac failure.

(11) *Cheyne-Stokes Respiration.* This is also known as periodic breathing. It is observed in normal individuals at very high altitudes and also in patients suffering from diseases affecting the circulation of the blood and the nutrition of the respiratory centre, heart disease, renal disease, cerebral conditions and in moribund patients.

An apnœic pause is followed by shallow respirations, which gradually increase in rate and depth until, reaching a maximum, they decrease again towards another period of apnœa; the whole cycle is then repeated. After several cycles the breathing may become normal again. Since it is a serious sign, it is important to note and report this phenomenon.

Asphyxia. This is the name given to the condition in which the normal exchange of gases between the atmospheric air and the body tissues is interrupted. It may be due to the lungs filling with water instead of air, as in drowning, or to poisonous gases being taken up by the blood instead of oxygen, *e.g.* coal gas. It also occurs where there is obstruction of the air passages, depression of the respiratory centre, paralysis of the respiratory muscles or when the tissues are unable to take up the oxygen from the blood, as in cyanide poisoning.

For the treatment of asphyxia see pages 339–349.

THE PULSE

The pulse is the wave of expansion felt in the elastic arteries when the heart pumps blood into vessels that, though always full, are distensible. The wave begins at the root of the aorta, gradually lessening as it spreads through the arterial system. In the capillaries there is normally no pulsation.

The pulse can be felt wherever a superficial artery runs over a bone, *e.g.* the radial, facial, temporal, posterior tibial and dorsalis pedis arteries. The most convenient site is usually the radial artery. The nurse should hold the patient's wrist on the palm of her hand and place her fingers along the course of the radial artery on the thumb side of the anterior surface of the wrist. The estimation of the rate should be made with the patient at rest. If he is not in bed, he should sit with the arm supported.

The nurse should accustom herself to the "feel" of the pulse before beginning to count the rate. An estimation of the force and rhythm of the beat should be made at the same time.

The Pulse Rate

The frequency of the heart beat is very constant in healthy persons in the resting state, but considerable individual variation may be found. It is usually said that the average rate in the adult is 72 per minute, but rates between 50 and 90 can be regarded as within the limits of the normal. It should be borne in mind, however, that for an individual who has a normal resting pulse rate of 60, a rate of 80 to 90 would be abnormal. In infancy the pulse rate is 120 to 140, at the age of three years about 100. In old age the rate tends to slow down.

Physiological Variations in the Normal Individual

Active muscular exercise may double the resting pulse rate, but there is quick return to normal after a short rest. Emotion also quickens the heart beat. These physiological increases enable the heart to increase its output per minute and so increase the blood supply to the working muscles. In the trained athlete, however, the heart responds to exercise with an increased strength of the beat without any great increase in rate. The heart beats more slowly in any condition in which the metabolic rate is decreased, *e.g.* complete rest, starvation.

Pathological Alterations in the Pulse Rate

Tachycardia. This is the term used to denote a quick action of the heart. The commonest conditions in which the rate is increased are:

(1) Fever, with the accompanying increased metabolic rate. The pulse rate usually rises 10 beats per minute for every $0.5°C$ ($1°F$) rise of temperature above $37.2°C$ ($99°F$).

(2) Increased activity of the thyroid gland (thyrotoxicosis).

(3) Lessened oxygen-carrying capacity of the blood in hæmorrhage and anæmia.

(4) Nervous disorder of the heart beat, paroxysmal tachycardia.

(5) A failing heart muscle; in any severe illness a rapid pulse which is also feeble is a very grave sign.

(6) Atrial (auricular) fibrillation uncontrolled by digitalis, when the pulse will be both rapid and irregular.

(7) The action of drugs, *e.g.* atropine, amyl nitrite.

Bradycardia. This means an excessively slow pulse and some of the commoner conditions in which this is found are:

(1) Stimulation of the vagus nerve due to increased intracranial pressure as a result of cerebral hæmorrhage, tumour or injury.

(2) Large dose of narcotic drugs, *e.g.* morphine.

(3) Disease of the conducting tissue of the heart leading to "heart block".

(4) Decreased activity of the thyroid gland, or any condition which markedly reduces the metabolic rate, for example extreme starvation.

Rhythm

Where any irregularity in rhythm is noted the pulse should be counted for a full minute; if it is counted for a quarter of a minute only there is greater opportunity for error. In all cases, too, where abnormal rhythm is noted the heart apex beat should be counted, using a stethoscope, and both rates should be charted. The apex beat can be located by placing the fingers over the fifth left intercostal space, slightly to the sternal side of the nipple line.

An entirely irregular pulse will show variations both in rhythm and in the strength of the beat. Some irregularities are transient and not important but when noted they should always be reported.

Sinus arrhythmia. This is a condition in which the pulse quickens on inspiration and slows on expiration. It may be noted in children and young adults and is of no significance.

Extra Systole. This is a condition in which the pulse is intermittent, an extra beat is followed by an abnormally long pause. The patient may be conscious of this and states that his heart "stops". In young people extra systoles are often due to irritation caused by excessive smoking, fatigue or a septic focus; in the older individual the condition is more likely to indicate some damage to the heart muscle.

Atrial (Auricular) Fibrillation. Fibrillation of the atria may occur in a number of cardiac conditions, such as mitral stenosis and coronary artery disease, and is also liable to occur in patients suffering from thyrotoxicosis. The atria have lost the power to contract rhythmically and a series of small contractions pass through the muscle continuously at the rate of about 450 per minute. Only some of these contractions stimulate the ventricles; nevertheless, although the ventricular rate is slower than the atrial rate, it will still be rapid, 200 or more per minute. Not all the ventricular contractions are strong enough to be transmitted to the radial artery and therefore the pulse rate will be less than the ventricular rate, this is known as the pulse deficit and is characteristic of atrial fibrillation. The ventricular rate may be 140 while the radial pulse rate is only 90 per minute, this is usually recorded as apex rate over pulse rate, $e.g.$ $\frac{140}{90}$; the difference between the two is pulse deficit; in this example it would be 50.

Digitalis is the drug most frequently employed in the treatment of atrial fibrillation; it may cause excessive slowing of heart rate and coupling of the pulse, in which two beats of unequal force are followed by an extra long pause. Slowing of the heart to a rate of less than 60 per minute from an initially high rate, $e.g.$ 180 per minute, is dangerous. It is therefore essential to check the rate and compare it with the previously recorded rate before giving the dose of digitalis; if the rate is falling rapidly no further dose should be given until this has been reported and medical advice has been sought.

BLOOD PRESSURE

Blood pressure is the force which the circulating blood exerts upon its enclosing walls and is maintained by:
    (1) the force of the ventricular contractions,
    (2) the state of the arterial walls,
    (3) the resistance in the arterioles,
    (4) the amount of blood in circulation.
The blood pressure must be maintained at a certain level to keep up the supply to the heart muscle and the vital centres in the brain. The average force of the pressure in the large arteries when the heart is actively pumping is sufficient to support a column of mercury 120 mm. high, and the average systolic pressure is said to be 120. The pressure when the heart is resting is about two-thirds of the systolic pressure: this is the diastolic pressure. The difference between the systolic and diastolic pressure gives the pulse pressure, $e.g.$ if the systolic pressure is 120 mm. of mercury and the diastolic pressure is 80 mm., the pulse pressure is 40 mm. The average range of the systolic pressure in an adult between 30 and 40 years old is 110 to 140 mm. In women the average pressure is 5 to 10 mm. lower than in men. At birth the average systolic

pressure is 30 to 40 mm. Other factors which affect the blood pressure are:

(1) Exercise and emotional excitement, which raise the pressure.

(2) Change of position. The pressure is lower in the recumbent than in the erect position.

A rise in pressure may be due to:

(1) Loss of elasticity of the vessel walls. Hardened arteries offer a greater resistance to the circulating blood and therefore the pressure rises. The condition commonly referred to as apoplexy, or a stroke, may result from rupture of vessels in the brain. Congestive heart failure may also result from the persistent extra burden on the heart.

(2) Fever. With a raised temperature and increased metabolism the pressure commonly rises, but with severe infection and marked toxæmia (*e.g.* diphtheria) the pressure may fall.

(3) Renal disease. A raised blood pressure may be present before renal efficiency tests or the presence of protein in the urine reveal diminished renal function.

A sustained rise in blood pressure with no discoverable cause is known as *essential hypertension*.

A fall in pressure may be due to:

(1) Surgical shock.

(2) Any sudden catastrophe, such as myocardial infarct.

(3) Severe loss of blood or plasma, or fluid through the gastrointestinal tract and as in persistent diarrhœa or vomiting.

(4) Adrenocortical insufficiency (Addison's disease).

(5) Sudden change in posture from the supine to the upright position; a fall in pressure from this cause is known as orthostatic hypotension.

When a serious and sudden fall in the blood pressure occurs the patient should immediately lie flat with the head low and the trunk and legs raised in order to maintain the blood supply to the vital centres in the brain. Subsequent treatment will depend on the cause of the condition.

Estimation of the Blood Pressure

Blood pressure is estimated with the apparatus known as a sphygmomanometer; it consists of a glass manometer containing

4

mercury and graduated in millimetres. An inflatable rubber cuff is attached by a piece of tubing to the manometer; this cuff is contained in a cotton bag so that when the inner rubber bag is inflated inside the cotton cover, it acts in the same way as a tourniquet and constricts the blood vessels in the arm to which it is applied. The cuff is fixed firmly and evenly round the patient's upper arm and is inflated by means of a small rubber hand pump. As the bag is inflated the column of mercury rises inside the manometer, the operator keeps his fingers over the patient's radial pulse and continues pumping until the pulse disappears. Then with a stethoscope placed over the brachial artery, which will be located above the elbow and on the inner side of the biceps muscle, the cuff is slowly deflated. The level at which tapping sounds, due to the returning pulse beat, can be heard is the level of the systolic pressure. With a further slow release of the pressure in the cuff all pulse sounds will disappear, the level of the mercury in the manometer at this point gives the diastolic reading.

When taking a patient's blood pressure he should be at rest, either sitting or lying down and his arm should be supported on the bed or on a table. Since strong emotion, such as fear, can affect the blood pressure a simple explanation should be given to the patient and he can be assured that the process is not painful. It is usually wise to keep the manometer turned away so that he cannot see the level of mercury during the procedure. The readings are usually recorded as systolic over diastolic pressure, *e.g.* $\frac{120}{80}$; alternatively they may be charted on a graph using two different coloured inks.

Charting

Making a chart is a graphic way of recording various data so that variations are readily appreciated by the eye.

It is the method by which variations in the temperature are most easily recorded, and the value of the chart is greatly increased if the pulse and respiratory rates and the blood pressure are also charted in the same way.

Where there is no reason to expect any sudden change in any of these signs a morning and evening chart is used. If there is fever, the temperature, pulse and respiration are recorded four-hourly. In certain cases hourly, half-hourly, or quarter-hourly charts of the pulse and/or blood pressure readings are kept.

INTAKE AND OUTPUT CHART

NAME _M. D. Brown_

DATE _10-1-62_   WARD _X.X._   CASE No.

TIME	IN		OUT				NOTES
	ORAL	INTRAVENOUS	ASPIRATION	URINE	VOMIT	DRAINAGE	
1 a.m	ml (CC)	1000 Dextrose/Saline ml (CC)	30 ml (CC)	ml (CC)	ml (CC)	ml (CC)	Clear fluid aspirated
2 a.m	Water 30 ml	ml	24 ml	200 ml	ml	ml	"
3 a.m	ml	ml	20 ml	ml	ml	ml	"
4 a.m	ml	ml	15 ml	ml	ml	ml	"
5 a.m	ml	ml	10 ml	ml	ml	ml	"
6 a.m	Water 30 ml	ml	20 ml	250 ml	ml	ml	"
7 a.m	ml	ml	36 ml	ml	ml	ml	"
8 a.m	Water 30 ml	ml	30 ml	ml	ml	ml	"
9 a.m	Water 30 ml	ml	36 ml	150 ml	ml	ml	"
10 a.m	Water 30 ml	1000 Dextrose 5% ml	24 ml	ml	ml	ml	"
11 a.m	Water 30 ml	ml	16 ml	ml	ml	ml	"
12 noon	Water 60 ml	ml	18 ml	360 ml	ml	ml	"
1 p.m	Water 60 ml	ml	20 ml	ml	ml	ml	"
2 p.m	Water 60 ml	ml	10 ml	ml	ml	ml	"
3 p.m	Water 60 ml	ml	24 ml	ml	ml	ml	"
4 p.m	Water 60 ml	ml	16 ml	500 ml	ml	ml	"
5 p.m	Water 60 ml	ml	18 ml	ml	ml	ml	"
6 p.m	Water 60 ml	ml	14 ml	ml	ml	ml	"
7 p.m	Water 60 ml	1000 Dextrose/Saline ml	10 ml	ml	ml	ml	"
8 p.m	Water 60 ml	ml	10 ml	460 ml	ml	ml	"
9 p.m	Water 60 ml	ml	12 ml	ml	ml	ml	"
10 p.m	ml	ml	ml	ml	ml	ml	—
11 p.m	ml	ml	10 ml	ml	ml	ml	Bile stained fluid
12 midn't	ml	ml	ml	ml	ml	ml	—
24 Hour Totals	780 ml	3000 ml	423 ml	1920 ml	ml	ml	

Na.	K.	Cl.	HCO₃	Hb			
							TOTAL **IN** 3780 ml
							TOTAL **OUT** 2343 ml
136-146 mEq/1	3.8-4.6 mEq/1	98-108 mEq/1	24-28 mEq/1				BALANCE 1437 ml

Fig. 8.1. INTAKE AND OUTPUT CHART.

A chart should be neatly and accurately kept and it is best to use a fine pen. Any written details should be in small but legible writing. The record of temperature, pulse and respiration, with notes on the action of the bowels, the quantity of urine passed, the amount of vomit or sputum, if any, are usually kept in a book and charted daily. Where a four-hourly chart is used the temperature, pulse and respiration should be charted as soon as taken. All special treatments and drugs are usually entered on the chart when given.

Records of the patient's fluid intake and fluid output are in many cases of great importance and the amounts are usually entered on a special form. The records should be made immediately whenever fluid is given and whenever fluid is lost by passing urine or by other routes, as for example by vomiting. The figures should be written in ordinary Arabic numerals, the use of Roman numerals may be a source of error, *e.g.* IX when written hurriedly may look very like IV, and in any case they are less quickly written and less easily read than the Arabic figures.

The aim in keeping a chart is to give as much information as possible regarding the patient's condition and treatment. The only permissible gaps in the temperature, pulse and respiration records are when the patient is sleeping and disturbance would be detrimental to his progress.

9 NUTRITION: FOOD AND FEEDING SICK PEOPLE

Increasing knowledge of the nutritional needs of the human body has done much to advance both curative and preventive medicine since the beginning of the present century. The essential requirements for a satisfactory diet for all human beings at all ages are adequate supplies of the body-building and energy-producing substances, proteins, carbohydrates, fats, and of the accessory substances, vitamins, mineral salts and water which are needed for the body fluids and for the regulations of cell metabolism. Most foods as commonly eaten contain a mixture of many of these substances; therefore, although the meals that the individual enjoys are very much a matter of personal taste and social custom, in favourable circumstances under-nutrition and nutritional disorders are rare in highly developed countries. In many parts of the world, however, poverty, ignorance, lack of natural resources, or disasters such as floods, drought or famine, may deprive large numbers of the population of the minimum food requirements for health.

Body-building and Energy-producing Foods

(1) **Proteins.** These are the foods required for growth and repair of the body tissues; they are also needed to supply the proteins in the blood plasma and for the production of enzymes, hormones, and antibodies. Protein in the diet in excess of these needs is used to produce heat and energy. Proteins are obtained from animal sources, meat, fish, eggs, cheese and milk and from vegetables such as cereals, peas, beans and nuts. The component units of the protein molecule are amino-acids; at least eight amino-acids are needed by the body cells and must be supplied in the diet. All of these eight are present in every one of the animal foods listed above, but any one of the vegetable sources will lack one or more of these essential substances. Proteins of animal

origin are therefore often described as "first class" and those obtained from vegetables as "second class" proteins. Everyone needs a daily protein intake of 1 g. per kilogram of body weight; children, pregnant women and nursing mothers will need proportionately more than those whose need is for maintenance and repair of tissue only. Most of us obtain our daily requirements of protein from both animal and vegetable foods. A strictly vegetarian diet necessitates the consumption of a considerable quantity of varied vegetable protein if the body's needs for all the amino-acids are to be met.

(2) **Carbohydrates.** These are the starches and sugars which when oxidized in the body provide heat and energy; carbohydrate in excess of the daily needs can be converted to fat and stored in the subcutaneous tissues and other "fat depots" of the body. Carbohydrates are necessary for the complete oxidation of fats; in their absence fats are not completely metabolized and ketone substances are produced which disturb the normal acid-base balance of the blood. Carbohydrates are obtained almost solely from vegetable sources (lactose in milk is one exception); very familiar examples are cereals, potatoes, root vegetables, fruits and the products obtained from these sources, *e.g.* bread, biscuits, jam and cane sugar. Vegetables and fruits contain a substance known as cellulose which cannot be digested in the human alimentary tract; this is useful in the normal diet as it provides a residual bulk in the large intestine which stimulates peristalsis and aids elimination.

(3) **Fats.** These foods come from animal sources, for example butter, cream, cheese, the fat of meat and some types of fish such as herrings, sardines and salmon, and from vegetables, mainly in the form of oils such as olive oil, sunflower seed oil, ground nut and palm nut oil; the nut oils are largely used in the manufacture of cooking fats and margarine. The metabolism of fats in the body provides heat and energy; fats also provide material for some of the body's secretions, such as sebum, and cholesterol and for protective coverings, such as the nerve sheaths.

Energy Requirements

The amount of energy resulting from the metabolism of proteins, carbohydrates and fats is measured in units known as

Calories. The "large calorie" used in dietetic calculations is the amount of heat required to raise the temperature of 1 kilogram of water 1°C.

Proteins when burnt as fuel have the same calorie value as carbohydrates, approximately 4 calories per gramme. The metabolism of fats yields rather more than double this value, approximately 9 calories per gramme.

Unless the diet is restricted for any reason, the average proportion of these body-building and energy foods in the daily diet is about 15 per cent. protein, 50 to 60 per cent. carbohydrate and 25 to 30 per cent. fat. Proteins and fats are more expensive than carbohydrates and therefore are liable to be replaced by excessive quantities of starches and sugars if money is short.

The daily requirements of the individual will vary with age, sex and occupation. An adult leading a moderately active life will need between 2,400 and 3,000 calories per day; a man undertaking strenuous physical work may require 4,000 calories or more. Children need more than might appear appropriate to their size; a child age 10 needs as much as a moderately active adult.

Vitamins

Vitamins are substances essential for life and health which are obtained from a wide variety of foods but which the body cannot, except in a few cases, manufacture itself. Vitamins found in fatty foods are classed as fat-soluble; these are vitamins A, D, E and K. The others are water-soluble and in this group are the numerous vitamins of the B complex and vitamin C.

Vitamin A promotes growth and is also needed for the protection of surface tissues and for the visual purple in the eye. It is present in animal tissues, fish liver oils, butter and cheese; in a partly-formed state, carotene, it is found in the pigment of vegetables such as carrots and tomatoes.

Vitamin B complex covers a number of substances, vitamin B_1 (thiamine or aneurine), riboflavine, nicotinic acid, B_{12} (cyanocobalamin), folic acid, pyrodixine, biotin and pantothenic acid. These vitamins are necessary for metabolism; folic acid and cyanocobalamin both prevent certain types of anæmia.

Vitamin C, or ascorbic acid, is present in many vegetables. It is easily destroyed by heat, but good sources are the citrus fruits, such as oranges, which are commonly eaten raw. Vitamin C is necessary for the normal growth of bones and teeth and for intercellular material such as the "cement" between the cells in the walls of the capillary blood vessels.

Vitamin D, calciferol, is found in milk, butter, fish and fish-liver oils such as halibut- and cod-liver oils. In the United Kingdom vitamin D is added to margarine. This vitamin is necessary for the growth and repair of bone and the proper development of teeth.

Vitamin E is found in milk, wheat germ and green vegetables. It has been found to influence fertility in experimental animals but there is no evidence that it has the same influence on human beings.

Vitamin K is found in most green vegetables and is an essential factor in the normal clotting of blood. The presence of bile in the small intestine is necessary for the absorption of vitamin K.

Mineral Salts

Mineral salts are inorganic substances present in a great many every day foods. The most important elements which the body obtains from mineral salts contained in food are calcium, phosphorus, sodium, potassium, iron, copper and iodine.

Calcium is found in milk, cheese, flour and green vegetables. In England calcium is added to all types of flour except wholemeal flour. Calcium is needed for the growth and repair of bone, and normal development of teeth. It is also one of the constituents in the blood plasma essential for the clotting of blood. Calcium is incompletely utilized in the absence of vitamin D.

Phosphorus is found in the same foods as calcium. It is required for the building of bones and teeth and for the normal functioning of the tissue cells.

Sodium is present in many foods and is also added to food in cooking or at the table in the form of common salt, sodium chloride. Sodium is present in the tissue cells and in the body fluids.

Potassium like sodium is found in a number of common food stuffs and it too is an essential constituent of the cells.

Iron is found in meat, eggs, whole grain bread and many vegetables. Iron is necessary for the hæmoglobin in the red blood cells and although the daily requirement of iron is small, if it is not met iron deficiency anæmia results.

Copper in the very small quantities required is not likely to be deficient in an ordinary mixed diet. This mineral is used in the formation of hæmoglobin.

Iodine is present in sea fish and in vegetables grown in soil containing iodine. It is needed, but again in small amounts only, for the manufacture of thyroxine in the thyroid gland.

Water

Water is essential for all living cells and for the various body fluids and secretions. The fluid requirements of the human body are discussed in Chapter 20 "Fluid and Electrolyte Balance".

FEEDING PATIENTS IN HOSPITAL

Patients' diets in hospital, other than those ordered individually from the special diet kitchen, are often classed as "full", "light" and "fluid". A patient taking full diet usually has three main meals, breakfast, midday dinner and supper, and the food served will be similar to that which he is accustomed to eat at home. Apart from therapeutic diets, some special diets may be needed for patients whose racial or religious customs may prohibit the eating of certain foods, for example, the kosher diet of the Jewish people and strictly vegetarian diets. Light diet commonly includes eggs, fish and chicken with additional milk drinks between main meals. Fluid diets, of which the basis is usually milk and sweetened fruit drinks, are generally served at two-hourly intervals.

Some of the difficulties encountered in catering for large numbers are the distances which the cooked food has to travel between the central kitchen and the wards and the need to cook some food a considerable time before it will be eaten. The proper planning of kitchens and the provision of adequate equipment helps to solve this latter problem. Trolleys with separate compartments for hot foods and for cold foods are in general use for the transport of food to the wards. More recently a tray system whereby individual meals are served directly on to the patient's trays in the kitchen and then conveyed immediately to the ward has been introduced in some hospitals. Special plates are used to keep hot food at the right temperature (Fig. 9.1).

Most hospitals have a catering committee which considers all aspects of providing food for patients and staff, buying supplies, approving dietary scales and arrangements for cooking and

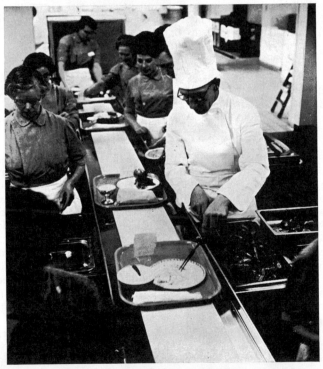

(*Radiography*)

Fig. 9.1. A MODERN CAFETERIA SYSTEM.

serving meals. Special therapeutic diets, for example diabetic, reducing or low calorie, high protein, calcium balance diets, are planned and supervised by a qualified dietitian.

Serving Meals

The nurse's part in the food service of the hospital is an important one as she is usually the person who presents it to the patient. It is essential that hot meals should be conveyed to the ward and served with the minimum of delay. All trays should be set beforehand, the kitchen prepared for this service and hot plates ready. Every nurse should consider it her responsibility to see that the best use is made of the food sent to the ward. If some simple cookery, such as boiling eggs for patients' breakfasts, is expected of her she should take a pride in doing this well. The art of cutting thin bread and butter and attractive sandwiches is well worth acquiring. Quite apart from the question of the patient's enjoyment of his meal it is obvious that poor cooking and indifferent service will result in considerable food wastage.

Food which looks tempting stimulates both the salivary and gastric secretion, so that digestion is aided. A badly served meal arouses a feeling of disgust, and the digestive functions are inhibited instead of helped. Unpleasant emotions such as fear or anger also destroy the appetite.

The tray and the tray cloth should be spotless. Glass and cutlery should be clean and shining.

All condiments allowed should be ready on the tray.

The patient's appetite should be taken into consideration; if it is small, only small portions should be served at first and a second helping offered. The tray should contain nothing that the patient is forbidden, and should not be crowded with unnecessary articles. If the patient can feed himself, he should be settled in a comfortable position and the tray placed where he can conveniently reach it.

Hot food must be really hot; hot drinks should be at the right temperature and not boiling. Cold food should be served cold and not tepid. Special feeds must be served punctually at the time ordered. Any complaints made by patients should at once be reported to the sister, and she should also be told if any patients have not eaten what was served.

Trays should be cleared away promptly and the crockery and cutlery neatly stacked in the kitchen ready for washing.

Feeding Helpless Patients

If a helpless patient has to be fed with a full diet he should be allowed time to eat properly, and not made to feel that the nurse is anxious for him to finish as quickly as possible. The patient should be supported in a comfortable position and the nurse should be seated at the right hand side of the bed facing the patient.

A helpless patient on a fluid diet is usually fed with a spouted feeder. The patient is told that he can control the flow of the liquid by putting his tongue over the opening of the spout; the feeder should be tilted sufficiently to allow him to get a good drink. If he is very weak, then he must be fed with small sips, and a spoon may be better than a feeding cup. The best method of supporting the patient's head while he drinks is to put an arm under his pillow raising this and the patient's head together.

Children who have not been trained to eat properly may require a great deal of kind, but firm, supervision at meal times. The nurse should not deal too firmly with a sick child who has developed many likes and dislikes over his food, but during a long stay in hospital the nurses can do a great deal to instil good habits into the child. If he can feed himself, it is usually better to let him do so, but his gown should be protected by a bib and the sheet by a cloth. Children as a rule demand frequent drinks of water, and in most cases this want should be satisfied. Sweets and fruit are best given after meals, and extra articles of food brought in should be given into the charge of the ward sister.

Special Difficulties

Feeding patients following injuries or operations on the mouth and tongue often calls for special care and management. Examples of such conditions which are fairly commonly seen, are harelip and cleft palate in infants and operations for malignant disease of the tongue.

(1) **Harelip Deformity.** Infants with this type of congenital deformity may be able to suck naturally, but if the condition of complete cleft palate is also present he will need to be fed with a

spoon or by an intragastric tube (see Chapter 18). For spoon feeding the child should be laid flat on the lap of the nurse or mother and the feed should be spooned into the hollow of the cheek, well to the back of the mouth. After operation for the repair of the lip, spoon feeding is continued using a small, narrow spoon which will not stretch the mouth. Crying will put additional strain on the stitches and it is therefore important that the infant should have adequate nourishment and fluid so that he does not cry from hunger or thirst. Water is given before and after each milk feed.

(2) **Cleft Palate Operation.** After this operation, which is usually performed at a later age than the repair of the harelip, but before the child begins to talk, feeding may be given by an intragastric tube or from a spouted feeding cup with a rubber tube attached. Cold liquids are usually given for the first few days, later semi-fluid feeds and soft solids given by spoon are allowed. A drink of water should be given before and after each feed to clean the mouth.

(3) **Operations on the Tongue** (including the insertion of radium needles). Following operation the patient is given a fluid diet either by an intragastric tube or from a spouted feeding cup with a rubber tube attached. The tubing should be put at the side of the mouth well to the back. Gentle irrigation of the mouth is usually ordered before and after feeds. If radium needles have been inserted their presence and position must be checked at the end of any treatment. Careful attention should be paid to thorough cleansing of the feeding cup and tubing after use, using a bottle brush for the spout and tubing. The cup and the rubber tubing should then be boiled and placed in a sterile covered bowl in readiness for the next feed.

Infant Feeding

The natural food for the new-born infant is the secretion of the mother's mammary glands. The breasts first secrete a substance called colostrum which contains some protein. On the third day after delivery milk is produced; human milk contains the proteins lactalbumin and casein, carbohydrate (in the form of lactose) and fat. This milk also contains protective antibodies which give the new-born infant a degree of immunity to certain infections.

It is generally accepted that every infant should be breast fed, at least for the first few weeks of his life, unless there is some contra-indication such as active tuberculosis in the mother.

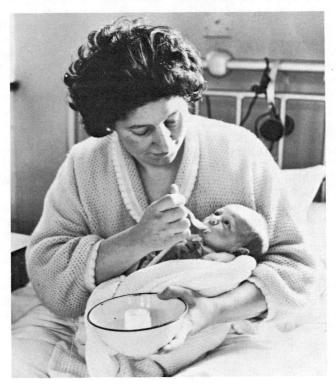

Fig. 9.2. SPOON FEEDING A NEW-BORN INFANT.

Many pædiatricians, however, now hold that the infant can and should have additions to this food at an early age, some say from birth. The infant's diet may therefore include pounded meat, and fish, eggs, cereals, sieved fruits and vegetables; also given are cow's milk, fruit juices and, of course, water to drink. With this type of diet a feeding bottle can be dispensed with, since the infant, apart from feeding at the breast, takes all his food from a spoon or cup. A mixed diet will usually provide the necessary vitamins; if the infant is fed on milk only, it is necessary to give orange or blackcurrant juice and fish-liver oil daily to ensure a sufficiency of vitamins C, A and D, since the vitamin content of both human and cow's milk is variable.

When an infant is admitted to hospital his feeding should if possible continue on the lines to which he is accustomed. His condition may, however, make this impossible. Milk is usually the basis of the feeds for a sick infant unable to take a mixed diet. Some addition, such as Farex two teaspoonfuls, or one table-spoonful of Benger's Food to one pint of milk, may be suitable.

The management of feeding difficulties in young infants and premature babies is a specialized subject on which the student is advised to consult a text book of pædiatric nursing.

When feeding an infant either with a spoon or a feeding bottle, the nurse or the mother should sit in a comfortable position with the child in her lap supported on her left arm. A sick baby may have to be fed in his cot. If a feeding bottle is used, it may be either the upright or the boat-shaped variety; the latter has two openings with a rubber valve at one end and a teat at the other; the upright bottle has only one opening, which is usually kept covered with a rubber cap which is exchanged for the feeding teat immediately before giving the feed. The hole in the teat should be large enough to allow the fluid to drop through, but not big enough to allow the infant to gulp the feed too quickly.

After use the bottle should be well flushed through with cold water then washed in warm soapy water and either boiled or autoclaved, or completely immersed in a tank of solution such as Milton 1 in 80. Teats are cleaned first in cold water, then in hot water and are then kept in a small covered jar containing Milton 1 in 80 until required. Salt rubbed over both inside and outside surfaces of the teat will remove grease when necessary. Teats may be boiled, but repeated boiling tends to soften the rubber.

Invalid Cookery

Cooking food increases its digestibility and improves and develops the flavour, thereby stimulating appetite; it destroys bacteria and parasites, and delays the putrefactive processes.

Food for invalids should be fresh and of the best quality obtainable. Variety should as far as possible be introduced, and the individual likes and dislikes of patients studied. It should be cooked in the simplest and most digestible ways, these are steaming, boiling, grilling or baking. As a general rule highly seasoned dishes and fried food are unsuitable. Meat, fish and eggs should not be overcooked, as the protein becomes hard and difficult to digest. Starchy foods are rendered more easily digestible by prolonged cooking.

BARLEY WATER (1)

Ingredients: 2 tablespoonfuls of pearl barley.
1 lemon.
2 tablespoonfuls of sugar.
2 pints water.

Method. Wash the barley and put in the saucepan with the thinly peeled rind of the lemon. Simmer gently for one and a half to two hours. Strain and add the lemon juice and sugar. Grape fruit may be used instead of lemon.

BARLEY WATER (2)

A quick method which makes a thinner drink may be preferred by many patients.

Method. The barley and lemon rind are placed in a warm jug and one pint of boiling water is added. The jug is covered and left to cool. Lemon juice and sugar are added to taste.

IMPERIAL DRINK

Ingredients: 1 teaspoonful of cream of tartar.
3 to 4 oz. sugar.
Juice of 1 lemon.
1 pint boiling water.

Method. Put the cream of tartar, sugar and lemon juice in a jug. Pour on the boiling water and stir well. Cover and use cold, diluting with plain water, barley water or soda water.

Milk Vegetable Soup

Ingredients: ½ pint milk.

Small piece of carrot, onion, celery and lettuce (if available) and turnip.

½ oz. butter.

½ oz. flour, lightly seasoned.

2 tablespoonfuls of cream if desired.

Method. Peel turnip, scrape carrot, skin onion, cut vegetables into fine shreds, sauté them in the butter in a saucepan (do not let them take colour), sprinkle in seasoned flour and cook. Add milk gradually, and bring to simmering point. Cook about twenty minutes, or until vegetables are tender. Serve very hot, with toast.

Baked Custard

Ingredients: 1 egg.

½ pint milk.

1 dessertspoonful of sugar.

Method. Grease the pie dish. Beat the egg and add the sugar and milk warmed, and pour into the pie dish. Place in a tin of cold water in the middle of a warm oven and allow to cook slowly, raising to the top shelf to brown.

Egg Jelly

Ingredients: ½ pint of liquid made up of the strained juice of 1 lemon and water.

Peel of 1 lemon thinly cut.

2 oz. loaf sugar, or to taste.

1 egg.

¼ oz. gelatin.

Method. Put all ingredients except the egg into a lined saucepan. Beat the egg and add, beating all the time. Stir over a very low heat with a fork until the gelatine is dissolved. The mixture *must not boil or it will curdle*. Cool, strain, mould, and when set turn out on to a small dish.

ORANGE JELLY

Ingredients: $\frac{1}{2}$ pint of liquid consisting of juice of 2 oranges
and 1 lemon.
$\frac{1}{4}$ oz. gelatin.
Rind of 1 orange and $\frac{1}{2}$ lemon thinly cut.
2 oz. of sugar.

Method. Put all the ingredients into a lined saucepan. Stir over a very gentle heat until the gelatin is dissolved. Cool, strain and mould.

BREAD AND BUTTER PUDDING

Ingredients: $1\frac{1}{2}$ gills milk.
1 egg.
1 dessertspoonful of sugar.
1 tablespoonful of clean sultanas.
2 or 3 slices (thin) of bread and butter.

Method. Grease pie dish well. Beat egg and milk together. Place bread and butter in dish (butter side downwards), sprinkle sultanas over, then add another layer of bread and butter. Pour custard over; stand aside for $\frac{1}{2}$ hour. Grate nutmeg over, if liked. Stand in tin of water; bake slowly until custard is set and the top a pale brown. Serve immediately.

SCRAMBLED EGGS

Ingredients: 1 or 2 new-laid eggs.
1 dessertspoonful of milk (for 2 eggs).
Piece of butter (size of walnut).
Slice of hot buttered toast.
Pepper and salt.

Method. Make toast, butter it and keep hot. Beat eggs a little with milk. Add pepper and salt. Melt butter in saucepan, pour in egg mixture, and cook slowly, stirring well until the egg is nearly set. Pile upon toast; garnish with parsley. Serve at once.

JUNKET

Ingredients: ½ pint milk.
Essence of rennet (quantity according to instructions on bottle).
1 teaspoonful of castor sugar.
Nutmeg or other flavouring, if desired.

Method. The junket bowls must be dry. Dissolve the sugar in the milk, making the milk luke-warm (temperature 98° to 100°F). Add the rennet and pour into junket bowls. Grate the nutmeg over the milk and leave until set.

STEAMED WHITING AND PARSLEY SAUCE

Method. Fillet and skin fish when necessary. Lay on board, skinned side up, season, squeeze a few drops of lemon juice over and roll up. Grease a soup plate, place the fish on the plate and cover with a greased paper and a saucepan lid. Place over a saucepan of boiling water; cook for about twenty minutes. Liquid from the fish should be used for the sauce, making up the required quantity of fluid with milk.

Sauce

Ingredients: ½ oz. butter.
½ oz. flour.
7 oz. liquid (milk, or milk and liquid from fish).
1 teaspoonful of chopped parsley.

Method. Melt the butter in a small saucepan. Remove from the heat and stir in the flour. Return the saucepan to the gas and cook slowly for about six minutes, but do not brown. Add the liquid slowly, beating well until free from lumps. Boil for eight minutes. Add the chopped parsley. Coat the fish and serve.

HIGH PROTEIN DRINKS

Used to increase the protein content of the diet as for example in the treatment of malnutrition, the nephrotic syndrome and extensive burns.

Ingredients: 10 oz. milk.
3 oz. dried skim milk.
$\frac{1}{2}$ oz. soluble protein (casein).
8 oz. water.

Protein value, 55 grammes;
Calorie value, 540.

Method. Measure the milk into a china bowl and whisk in the dried skim milk and the soluble protein. Add the water and strain. The drink may be served warm or cold sweetened and flavoured according to taste with coffee, cocoa, etc. The mixture must not be boiled as this will coagulate the soluble protein.

A proprietary preparation, Complan, is a convenient and palatable high protein drink, which is often found useful in the dietetic treatment of peptic ulcers and ulcerative colitis. 100 grammes of Complan contains 31 grains of protein, 16 grammes of fat and 44 grammes of carbohydrate with an energy value of 450 calories. Complan is supplied as a powder which dissolves readily in hot or cold water or in milk.

10 ADMINISTRATION OF DRUGS: WEIGHTS AND MEASURES: SOLUTIONS: THERMOMETRIC SCALES

Drugs are substances obtained from vegetable, mineral and animal sources and used for medicinal purposes. They may be introduced into the body in various forms and by various routes. Drugs may be dispensed in liquid form as solutions, tinctures, infusions, emulsions or oils, or in solid form as pills, powders, tablets or capsules.

Drugs may be administered by mouth, occasionally by the rectum, or parenterally, that is to say they may be introduced by other routes than the alimentary tract, such as subcutaneous, intramuscular or intravenous injections, or by inhalation.

Medicines for administration by mouth must be stored in a cupboard reserved for this purpose, and substances intended for external application only must be kept in a separate cupboard.

Drugs controlled by the Dangerous Drugs Act

The Dangerous Drugs Act controls the sale and use of substances liable to cause drug addiction. Opium and its alkaloids, notably morphine, cocaine and Indian hemp were the drugs controlled by the original Act; more recent additions are pethidine hydrochloride, methadone hydrochloride (Physeptone) and phenadoxone hydrochloride (Heptalgin). These drugs may be supplied to the public only on the written prescription of a medical practitioner. Hospital wards and departments are, however, authorized to keep a stock of certain preparations, such as morphine and pethidine, but they must be ordered on a duplicate form signed by the authorized responsible person, *i.e.* the sister or charge nurse who is responsible for the safe storage of the drugs and for ensuring that they are used only in accordance with written orders of the medical staff. D.D.A. drugs must be kept in a locked cupboard reserved for the storage of these drugs the key of which is kept by the sister or charge nurse; the containers must have the words "D.D.A." written on the label. All prescriptions and order forms must be kept by the hospital for a period of two years from the date of issue.

The Poisons and Pharmacy Act

The Poison and Pharmacy Act controls the sale, prescription and use of a very large range of substances which are potentially toxic or dangerous. There are sixteen schedules under the Act which list a great number of poisonous substances and the regulations to be observed in their use. The two schedules which are of particular importance in medical and hospital practice are the First and Fourth Schedules.* In hospitals Schedule I can be considered as including Schedule IVA drugs; they can be obtained from the pharmacist's department only on the written order of a medical officer or the sister or charge nurse of the ward or department. They must be clearly labelled Schedule I and stored in a locked cupboard. It should be noted that the toxic and addiction forming drugs controlled by the Dangerous Drugs Act are also listed on Schedule I. The usual practice with regard to storage is to have a drug cupboard for Schedule I poisons with an inner cupboard fitted with a separate lock and key for D.D.A. Drugs. It is important to remember that the "poisons cupboard" must be reserved solely for the storage of D.D.A. and Scheduled drugs.

Examples of drugs on the First and Fourth Schedules of the Poisons and Pharmacy Act are the toxic alkaloids such as atropine and hyoscine and the barbiturates.

Each ward and department should keep a Dangerous Drugs and Poisons record book in which the patient's name, the drug, the dose, the date and the time of administration are entered and each entry signed by the nurse giving and the nurse checking the drug.

The Therapeutic Substances (Prevention of Misuse) Act, 1956

The Therapeutic Substances Act controls substances which are capable of causing danger to the health of the community if used

---

* Schedule IV is now divided into Part A and Part B. Part A drugs are subject to the same controls as Schedule I drugs. Part B lists drugs which are to be used only on prescription and under medical supervision.

without proper safeguards. The form of prescription is the same as for Fourth Schedule Drugs which may only be prescribed by a medical practitioner, dentist or veterinary surgeon. Drugs controlled by this Act include antibiotics, cortisone, prednisone and isoniazid.

Administration of Drugs by Mouth

Rules. (1) Read the label on the bottle before removing the bottle from the shelf and again before pouring out the dose.

(2) Shake the bottle.

(3) Hold the bottle with the labelled side uppermost. A soiled label is not only unsightly, but dangerous, since it may become illegible.

(4) Remove the cork, holding it in the little finger of the left hand.

(5) Measure the dose at eye level.

(6) If there is a sediment, provide a glass rod to stir the medicine immediately before the patient takes it.

(7) Check once more to be sure that you have the right medicine, the right dose, and that you are taking it to the right patient.

(8) Give the medicine at the correct time and see that the patient takes it.

(9) If the mixture contains a drug controlled by the Dangerous Drugs Act or a Schedule I drug a second person should check the dose.

(10) Once poured out, the medicine should not be returned to the bottle. Medicine should never be given from an unlabelled or illegibly labelled bottle, or from an unmarked container.

Times for Administration of Medicine. If a medicine is ordered three times a day with no other directions, it is given immediately after the three main meals of the day, *i.e.* breakfast, dinner and supper.

A medicine ordered before food is given fifteen to twenty minutes before a meal.

A medicine ordered twice a day is usually given after breakfast and supper, unless special times are stated.

A medicine ordered four-hourly is given at four-hourly intervals throughout the day and night, but special instructions should be obtained regarding waking the patient at night.

Slow-acting purgatives are given at night, quick-acting purgatives in the early morning.

General Remarks. Many medicines have an unpleasant taste, and the majority of patients can be allowed a drink of water, a piece of fruit or a sweet to take away the taste.

Holding the nose while drinking is sometimes a help, as taste depends to some extent on smell.

A medicine containing iron, stains the teeth and should be taken through a glass drinking tube or a straw. The mouth should be washed out afterwards and the teeth cleaned.

Powders are most easily swallowed if put upon the tongue and washed down with a drink of water. They may be put into a rice-paper cachet, which should be moistened with some water in a spoon, as it can then be more easily swallowed.

Pills and capsules are swallowed with a drink of water.

Oily substances are difficult to take, not only on account of the flavour, but also because of the disagreeable taste of oil in the mouth. Liquid paraffin has no distinct flavour and is fairly easy to swallow if a little soda or plain water is added. Castor oil is extremely unpleasant to take, both on account of its taste and the thickness of the oil. Infants, however, will usually take castor oil from a spoon quite readily, and older children will often take it beaten up in warm milk. For an adult patient the oil must be prepared so that the patient can drink it all at once without tasting it. One method is to warm a china measure or medicine glass in hot water; about 2 teaspoonfuls of lemon juice or mixed lemon and orange juice are poured into the measure and the prescribed dose of the oil floated on top of this. More fruit juice is poured on to the top of the oil. A slice of lemon or orange may be taken to the bedside with the dose. The patient is told to bite the piece of lemon, then swallow the dose at one gulp and bite the slice of lemon again.

The disadvantages of giving drugs by mouth are:

(1) The patient may not be able or may refuse to swallow the dose.

(2) The drug may be only partially absorbed.

(3) It may irritate the alimentary tract, causing vomiting or acting as a purgative, so that the desired effect is lost.

Administration of Drugs by the Rectum

The drug is dissolved in about 120 ml. (4 oz.) of normal saline or water and injected slowly at body temperature.

Examples of drugs which may be given per rectum are potassium bromide, chloral hydrate and bromethol.

Parenteral Administration of Drugs

Hypodermic Injection

Hypodermic (or subcutaneous) injection is the method commonly used when it is desirable that the drug should act quickly, when only a small volume of fluid is to be injected and when the solution is not likely to damage the superficial tissues. Drugs which may be irritant in the subcutaneous tissue must be injected either into muscle, which has a good blood supply, or into a vein. It should also be noted that, if the superficial circulation is depleted, absorption of a substance injected hypodermically is likely to be slow and uncertain. Therefore morphine, for example, which is commonly given by hypodermic injection, may be given intravenously to a patient suffering from severe shock.

Drugs for hypodermic injection are usually dispensed in solution, either in single dose ampoules, which provide a considerable safeguard against accidental over-dosage, or in multidose containers. Tablets which are dissolved in sterile water immediately before use are also obtainable and, although not often seen in hospitals now, they may be used in private practice. The usual sites for injection are the outer aspect of the upper arm or the thigh.

Syringes of 1 or 2 ml. capacity are used, with size 17 to 20 needles (for sterilization of syringes see pages 136–139. Before giving the injection the nurse must make sure that the needle is not bent or blunt. A bent needle may snap during the injection, a blunt needle will cause the patient unnecessary pain. Where a central service deals with all syringes and needles, every needle is inspected and sharpened after each use. "Disposable" needles, used for one injection only, are supplied in some hospitals.

If a syringe has been stored in alcohol this must be expelled and the syringe washed in sterile water before use.

The nurse should place the syringe on a tray, with the needle resting on a piece of sterile gauze, together with a swab moistened with alcohol or cetrimide for cleaning the skin. A pair of sterile dressing forceps for handling the needle may be required. She should take the tray with the bottle or container and the patient's prescription sheet to a second person to be checked. The dose should be measured in the presence of the person checking it.

Solutions for hypodermic injections may be dispensed in multidose rubber-capped bottles. The bottle should be held so that the cap is not handled. After wiping the cap of the bottle with a swab moistened with alcohol, the needle should be pushed through the centre of the cap and a little air injected to facilitate the removal of the fluid. Slightly more than the required quantity of the solution should be taken up, and then, holding the syringe with the needle vertical, the piston is pushed up until the edge is on a level with the line showing the required number of minims.

When using drugs in tablet form a small amount of water should be boiled in a spoon and a convenient amount, 0·5 to 1 ml. (10 to 15 minims) taken up in the syringe. The excess water in the spoon is then discarded, the tablet placed in the spoon, and the water from the syringe expelled into it. The tablet dissolves readily and the solution is drawn up into the syringe.

If the drug is in a glass ampoule, a file is required to make a mark on the neck of the ampoule where it is to be broken. The outside of the glass is washed with a swab, moistened with alcohol and, holding the ampoule in a piece of sterile gauze, the neck is then broken at the file mark.

If the patient is not familiar with the procedure, the nurse should explain to him what she is about to do and that he will feel only a very small prick. An injection made with a sharp needle is scarcely felt.

The site of the injection should be rubbed fairly vigorously with a swab moistened with alcohol, in order both to cleanse the skin and to increase the blood supply. A small piece of skin and subcutaneous tissue should be taken up between the thumb and first finger of the left hand, pulling the skin fairly taut. The needle is inserted quickly and firmly into the fold of subcutaneous tissue, and the piston pushed steadily down. The mop should be pressed on the skin while the needle is withdrawn.

Among the drugs commonly given by hypodermic injection are adrenaline, atropine, hyoscine, morphine, papaveretum (Omnopon) and nikethamide (Coramine).

Intramuscular Injection

This method is used when larger amounts are required to be injected than can be given by hypodermic injection, and is also chosen when the drug would be irritating if injected superficially. The sites usually chosen are the vastus externus muscle of the outer aspect of the thigh, the gluteal muscles of the buttock, or the deltoid muscle in the upper part of the arm (Fig. 10.1). It is essential

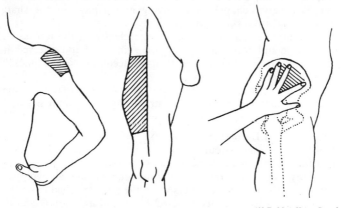

(*N.E. Met. Hosp. Board*)

Fig. 10.1. THREE SITES FOR INTRAMUSCULAR INJECTIONS.
Left: Outer Aspect of the Shoulder.
Centre: Antero-lateral Aspect of the Thigh.
Right: Anterior Part of the Upper and Outer Quadrant of the Buttock.

to avoid giving the injection into a blood vessel, nerve or periosteum. To ascertain that the needle is not in a vein the plunger should be withdrawn a little; if blood is drawn up into the syringe, then a vein has been punctured and the needle should be moved slightly and the plunger once more withdrawn before making the injection. When making an injection into the buttock the upper and outer quadrant should be chosen, as there is a risk of stabbing the sciatic nerve if the needle is inserted too near the sacrum. The periosteum can be avoided by giving the injection into a site where there is plenty of muscle covering the bone and by not stabbing too deeply.

The injection and the skin over the site are prepared in the manner described for the giving of hypodermic injections. The size of syringe and needles required will depend on the amount and type of the drug to be injected and on the site of the injection, 1, 2 or 5 ml. syringes may be needed and needles 2 to $2\frac{1}{2}$ inches long.

The needle should be long enough to penetrate the muscle without inserting it up to the mount as, should the needle break, there is a better chance of removing it if a piece of the shaft projects above the skin surface.

The skin over the selected site is stretched with the left hand. The syringe and needle are held in the right hand and directed at a right angle to the skin surface, then the needle is inserted quickly and firmly deep into the muscle.

Many drugs may be given by intramuscular injection. Some common examples are penicillin, streptomycin, vitamin B_{12} and Imferon.

Sensitization Dermatitis. Dermatitis, particularly of the hands, arms and face, may occur in nurses and doctors who come into frequent contact with penicillin and streptomycin when giving injections. An investigation into this problem has shown that spraying of the antibiotic occurs when the air is expelled from the syringe and when the needle used for withdrawal of the drug from the container is changed for another needle for giving the injection. Contamination of the hands is also likely if there is a leakage at the junction of the needle and the nozzle of the syringe. In order to minimize the risk of dermatitis it is recommended that the air should be expelled from the syringe into the container before the needle is withdrawn and that the same needle should be used for giving the injection. Care should also be taken to ensure that the needle is firmly attached to the syringe. Wearing rubber gloves gives added protection and the gloves, hands and arms should be thoroughly washed under running water when the procedure is completed. The syringe and needle should also be washed under running water.

Prolonged testing has proved that the needle is not blunted by puncturing the rubber cap of the container.

Disposable Injection Units. Disposable drug containers and injectors are available which have the advantages of providing sealed sterile equipment ready for immediate use. The use of these injector units for antibiotic drugs reduces the risk of sensitization dermatitis for doctors and nurses who have to give large numbers of these injections. The apparatus consists of a glass ampoule

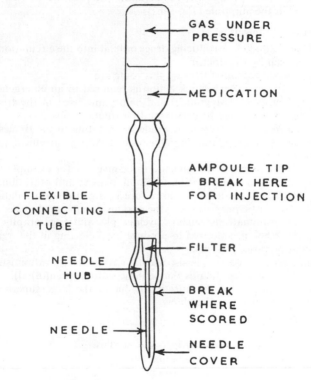

Fig. 10.2. An Automatic Injector.

(Adapted from *Emergencies in Medical Practice*, by courtesy of E. & S. Livingstone Ltd.)

containing the solution to be injected, an inert gas and a needle protected by a glass sheath. A flexible plastic tube covers the neck of the ampoule and the mount of the needle. When using the injector the glass sheath is given a quick snap and removed, the needle is then inserted into the tissues and the flexible tube squeezed and released. If the needle has entered a vein blood will be seen on the filter pad round the needle. If no blood appears the neck of the ampoule is broken by bending the plastic tube and the solution flows through the needle under the pressure exerted by the gas in the ampoule (Fig. 10.2).

Intravenous Injection

This method of introducing drugs or fluid into the circulation is undertaken by the doctor.

The usual reasons for using this route are:

(1) When a very quick action is required in an emergency, *e.g.* bemegride (Megimide) and nalorphine used in the treatment of coma due to poisoning by narcotic drugs.

(2) When the drug used would be irritating to the tissues if given intramuscularly or hypodermically, *e.g.* arsenical preparations.

(3) When large amounts are to be given as for example the intravenous administration of blood, plasma and other fluids.

(4) When it is desired to introduce a drug into the circulation for diagnostic purposes, *e.g.* the various opaque media used in X-ray examinations, such as pyelography and angiography.

(5) When it is desired to produce local clotting in the treatment of varicose veins.

Intravenous injection is also used as a route for the administration of anæsthetics such as thiopentone sodium (Pentothal).

The usual site for the injection is one of the large superficial veins on the front of the elbow.

Requirements:

The drug for injection.

A sterile 10 or 20 ml. syringe and needles.

A tourniquet or a sphygmomanometer.

A roller bandage for the patient to grip.

Sterile swabs and a sterile towel.

Instrument forceps.

Ether, surgical spirit or cetrimide.

A mackintosh.

A small gauze dressing and collodion for sealing the puncture.

A receiver for dirty swabs.

The skin should be cleaned round the site of the injection, and the tourniquet or the cuff of the sphygmomanometer placed round the arm well above the elbow and then tightened or inflated sufficiently to distend the veins. The cuff of the sphygmomanometer is more convenient than a tourniquet, as it is easier to regulate the pressure so that the venous, but not the arterial, circulation is stopped. Also the wide cuff of the sphygmomanometer is more comfortable for the patient than a narrow rubber tourniquet.

The patient, if able to do so, may help by gripping the roller bandage tightly or by opening and closing his fist several times.

The nurse will be required to assist by steadying the patient's arm while the needle is being inserted and by releasing the tourniquet or deflating the cuff when the needle is in the vein.

Inhalation

Drugs given by inhalation may be used for their general effect, or for their local action on the respiratory tract. The substances used must be either in the form of a vapour, or a liquid which readily vaporizes, or a fine spray, such as an aerosol spray. The anæsthetic gases are examples of drugs exerting a general effect when inhaled. Aromatic substances, such as menthol and tincture of benzoin, may be added to steam inhalations for their local effect in the treatment of upper respiratory infections such as acute sinusitis and laryngitis. The administration of antibiotics by aerosol inhalation is occasionally ordered in the treatment of certain lung infections and an aerosol spray of an antispasmodic drug, isoprenaline, may be ordered in the treatment of asthma.

WEIGHTS AND MEASURES
Metric System
Measures of Mass (Weights)

1 milligram (mg.) $=\frac{1}{1000}$ gramme or 0·001 g.
1 centigram (cg.) $=\frac{1}{100}$ gramme or 0·01 g.
1 decigram (dg.) $=\frac{1}{10}$ gramme or 0·1 g.
1 gramme (G. or g.) = weight of 1 millilitre (ml.) of distilled water at 4°C. The accepted symbol in prescription writing is G., since gm. and grm. are likely to be confused with gr. (grain).
1 kilogram (kg.) = 1,000 grammes.

Measures of Capacity (Volumes)

1 centimil (cml.) = the vol. of 1 centigram of water at 4°C.
1 decimil (dml.) = the vol. of 1 decigram of water at 4°C.
1 millilitre
  or mil (ml.)   = the vol. of 1 gramme of water at 4°C.
1 litre (l.)   = the vol. of 1,000 grammes (1 kg.) of water at
                 4°C.

N.B.—The cubic centimetre (c.c.), which is approximately equal to 1 millilitre, should not be used as a unit of volume. The accepted abbreviation for "millilitre" is "ml."

Imperial System

Measures of Mass (Weights)

Apothecaries'
  1 grain (gr.)
  1 scruple = 20 grains.
  1 drachm = 60 grains = 3 scruples.
  1 ounce = 480 grains = 8 drachms.
  1 pound (lb.) = 12 ounces = 5,760 grains.

Avoirdupois
  1 grain (gr.)
  1 ounce (oz.) = 437·5 grains.
  1 pound (lb.) = 16 ounces = 7,000 grains.

Measures of Capacity (Volumes)

  1 minim (m.)
  1 fluid drachm (fl. dr.) = 60 minims.
  1 fluid ounce (fl. oz.) = 8 fl. dr.
  1 pint   = 20 fl. oz.
  1 quart   = 2 pints.
  1 gallon   = 4 quarts.

Roman numerals were formerly used in prescription writing, *e.g.* I, II, III, IV. It is now recommended that Roman numerals and the ancient symbols (*e.g.* ℨ, ℥) be no longer used, and that quantities ordered should be written in arabic numerals and expressed in simple abbreviations—*e.g.* grains (gr.), ounces (oz.), fluid ounces (fl. oz.), drachms (dr.), minims (m.).

Approximate Equivalents—Imperial and Metric

Weight: Imperial to Metric

Imperial Grain	Metric Milligram	Imperial Grains	Metric Milligrams
$\frac{1}{600}$	0·1	$\frac{1}{4}$	15
$\frac{1}{200}$	0·3	$\frac{1}{3}$	20
$\frac{1}{100}$	0·6	$\frac{1}{2}$	30
$\frac{1}{60}$	1	$\frac{3}{4}$	50
$\frac{1}{50}$	1·25	1	60
$\frac{1}{40}$	1·5	$1\frac{1}{2}$	100
$\frac{1}{30}$	2	2	125
$\frac{1}{25}$	2·5	3	200
$\frac{1}{20}$	3	4	250
$\frac{1}{15}$	4	5	300
$\frac{1}{12}$	5	6	400
$\frac{1}{10}$	6	8	500
$\frac{1}{8}$	7·5	10	600
$\frac{1}{6}$	10	12	800
$\frac{1}{5}$	12·5	15	1000

$\frac{1}{2}$ oz. (Av.)	14·2 grammes
1 oz. (Av.)	28·35 ,,
1 pound (Av.)	453·6 ,,

Weight: Metric to Imperial

$$1 \text{ kilogram} = 2 \text{ lb. } 3\frac{1}{4} \text{ oz.}$$
$$500 \text{ grammes} = 1 \text{ lb. } 1\frac{1}{2} \text{ oz.}$$
$$100 \text{ grammes} = 3\frac{1}{2} \text{ oz.}$$
$$25 \text{ grammes} = \tfrac{4}{5} \text{ oz.} = 386 \text{ grains.}$$
$$10 \text{ grammes} = \tfrac{1}{3} \text{ oz.} = 154 \text{ grains.}$$
$$1 \text{ gramme} = 15\cdot4 \text{ grains.}$$
$$0\cdot5 \text{ gramme} = 7\cdot7 \text{ grains.}$$

5

Volume: Imperial to Metric

Minims	Millilitres		Fl. drachms	Millilitres
½	0·03		½	1·8
1	0·06		1	3·6
2	0·12		2	7·1
3	0·18		6	21·3
4	0·24			
5	0·3		Fl. ounces	Millilitres
6	0·4		½	14·2
8	0·5		1	28·4
10	0·6		2	56·8
12	0·7		4	113·7
15	0·9		5	142·1
20	1·2		6	170·5
25	1·5		8	227·5
30	1·8		10	284·2
40	2·4		20	568·4
45	2·7			
60	3·6		Gallons	Litres
90	5·3		1	4·546
120	7·1			
240	14·2			

Relations of Volume to Weight

1 minim is the volume at 16·7°C (62°F) of 0·911 grain of water.

1 fl. drachm is the volume at 16·7°C (62°F) of 54·687 grains of water.

1 fl. ounce is the measure at 16·7°C (62°F) of 437·5 grains of water. (Av. ounce.)

1 pint is the measure at 16·7°C (62°F) of 8750·0 grains of water.

Percentage Solutions

The term "per cent." is used to mean:

(a) Per cent. W/W = weight in weight.

(b)   ,,   ,,   V/V = volume in volume.

(c)   ,,   ,,   W/V = weight in volume.

Where the Imperial System of weights and measures is used, calculation of dosage presents a difficulty because 1 minim is not the volume of 1 grain of water but only of 0·911 grain. Therefore 100 grains of water measure 110 minims (accurately 109·7143) at 16·7°C. Therefore a 1 per cent. W/V solution equals 1 grain in 110 minims.

From above figures the amounts can be calculated for any quantity of a solution of any percentage.

1 per cent. solution prepared according to the metric system is equivalent to 1 gramme in 100 ml., and prepared according to the Apothecaries' System is equivalent to 1 grain in 110 minims.

The Metric System is increasingly used in prescribing and the dosage of most of the newer drugs is expressed in terms of this system. In giving approximately equivalent Metric and Imperial dosages it is usual to reckon that 1 gramme = 15 grains and 1 millilitre = 15 minims. 1 grain is taken to equal 60 milligrams.

Table of Percentage Solutions

(To nearest second decimal figure)

Per cent.	Grains per fl. oz.	Per cent.	Grains per fl. oz.
10·0	43·75	1·8	7·88
9·5	41·56	1·7	7·44
9·0	39·37	1·6	7·00
8·5	37·19	1·5	6·56
8·0	35·00	1·4	6·12
7·5	32·81	1·3	5·69
7·0	30·62	1·2	5·25
6·5	28·44	1·1	4·81
6·0	26·25	1·0	4·37
5·5	24·06	0·9	3·94
5·0	21·87	0·8	3·50
4·5	19·69	0·7	3·06
4·0	17·50	0·6	2·62
3·5	15·31	0·5	2·19
3·0	13·12	0·4	1·75
2·5	10·94	0·3	1·31
2·0	8·75	0·2	0·87
1·9	8·31	0·1	0·44

Method of Calculating Fractional Doses and of Diluting Stock Solutions

Many of the drugs given by parenteral routes, *i.e.* subcutaneously, intravenously and intramuscularly, are commonly dispensed in ampoules containing one therapeutic dose, *e.g.* morphine is dispensed in ampoules containing $\frac{1}{6}$, $\frac{1}{4}$, $\frac{1}{3}$ and $\frac{1}{2}$ grain. Drugs are, however, also dispensed in rubber-capped bottles of stock solution and it may be necessary to calculate a fractional dose from the solution supplied and examples of the method employed are, therefore, given:

Example. The solution of hyoscine hydrobromide supplied is $\frac{1}{160}$ gr. in 15 minims water and the prescribed dose for a patient is $\frac{1}{100}$ grain. $\frac{1}{160}$ gr. in 15 minims = 1 gr. in 160×15 minims. Therefore $\frac{1}{100}$ gr. will be contained in $\dfrac{160 \times 15}{100} = 24$ minims.

To Dilute Stock Solutions of Lotions. Divide the strength of the dilution required by the strength of the stock solution to obtain the total number of parts required; one part will be stock solution, the remaining number of parts the required addition of the diluent.

Example. Stock solution of lotion is 1–20 and 24 fl. oz. of a dilution of 1–120 is required.

120 divided by 20 = 6; therefore, 1 part of the 1–20 solution and 5 parts of water, *i.e.* 4 fl. oz. phenol and 20 fl. oz. water, are required.

Young's formula for calculating the proportion of the adult dose of a drug to be given to a child:

$$\left(\frac{\text{Age of child}}{\text{Age of child} + 12} \right) \times \text{adult dose.}$$

Example. The adult dose of a mixture containing bromide is 1 oz. How much of this mixture should be given to a child aged six?

$$\left(\frac{6}{6 + 12} \right) \times 480 \text{ minims—} i.e. \text{ 160 minims.}$$

Note. Young's formula is an approximation and should be used only with certain reservations. Dosage is more often calculated according to body weight.

Insulin Dosage

The standard strengths of insulin for injection are:

20 units per ml.
40 units per ml.
80 units per ml.

For the injection of insulin a syringe of 1 ml. capacity graduated in 20 divisions may be used and this is the type usually supplied to the patient who gives his own injections. If the insulin solution to be used is single strength, *i.e.* 20 units in each ml., then each division represents 1 unit, if it is double strength then each division is 2 units, and if it is quadruple strength each division is 4 units. Obviously the patient must be carefully instructed as to the exact amount to be drawn up into the syringe and this is particularly important if the dosage or the strength of the insulin is altered. For example, if the dose is 40 units and double strength insulin is used, then the patient must draw up 1 ml., 20 divisions; if, however, a change is made to quadruple strength and the dose remains at 40 units, then each division represents 4 units and the amount to be drawn is 0·5 ml., *i.e.* 10 divisions.

Syringes of 1 or 2 millilitre capacity are also used for the injection of insulin and these syringes may be graduated in 0·1 ml. ($\frac{1}{10}$) or 0·2 ml. ($\frac{1}{5}$).

Using a syringe in which each division on the barrel corresponds to 0·1 ml., and with an insulin strength of 20 units per ml., each division represents 2 units of insulin. If the strength of insulin is 40 units per ml. then each division represents 4 units of insulin, and with 80 units per ml. each division represents 8 units of insulin.

Examples. (1) The strength of the insulin to be used is 40 units per ml. and the dose ordered is 32 units.

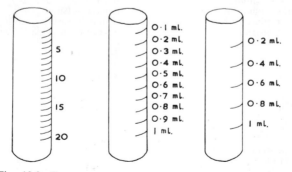

Fig. 10.3. Graduations on "Insulin" Syringe and 1 ml. Syringe Barrels.

The required dose will be $\frac{32}{40}$ ml. $= 0.8$ ml., and since each division on the syringe represents 4 units, the amount to be drawn up will correspond with the eighth graduation on the barrel ($\frac{32}{4} = 8$).

If each division on the syringe used represents 0·2 ml. then, using insulin in the strength of 20 units per ml., each graduation equals 4 units of insulin. If the insulin strength is 40 units per ml. each graduation equals 8 units, and with 80 units per ml. each graduation equals 16 units of insulin.

(2) Using a syringe graduated in 0·2 ml. and insulin in the strength of 80 units per ml., the dose ordered is 64 units.

The required dose will be $\frac{64}{80}$ ml. $= 0.8$ ml., and since each division on the syringe represents 16 units the amount to be drawn up will correspond with the fourth graduation on the barrel ($\frac{64}{16} = 4$).

Latin Words and Abbreviations used in Prescription Writing

Word or Abbreviation	*Meaning*
Aa, Ana (Greek preposition)	Of each.
Ad lib., Ad libitum	As much as is desired.
B.i.d., Bis in die	Twice a day.
B.P.	British Pharmacopœia.
c., Cum	With.
C., Congius	A gallon.
Cataplasma	A poultice.
Cibus	Food.
A.c., Ante cibum	Before food.
P.c., Post cibum	After food.
Collun, Collunárium	A nasal wash.
Collut., Collutorium	A mouth wash.
Collyr., Collyrium	An eye wash.
Co., Compositus	Compound.
Cras	Tomorrow.
Emplastrum	A plaster.
Flavus	Yellow.
*G., g.	Gramme.
gr., Granum, Grana	A grain, grains.
Gtt., Gutta, Guttæ	A drop, drops.
H., Hora	An hour.
Lb., libra	A pound.
Mane	In the morning.
Mist., Mistura	A mixture.
Mol., Mollis	Soft.

* Great care must be taken to distinguish between the symbols for a *gramme* and a *grain*; mistakes have been made by confusing "g" with "gr".

Nocte	..	..	..	..	At night.
O., Octarius	..	..	..	..	A pint.
Ol., Oleum	..	..	..	..	Oil.
Om., Omnis	..	..	..	..	All, every.
O.h., Omni hora	..	..	..	Every hour.
O.m., Omni mane	..	..	..	Every morning.
O.n., Omni nocte	..	..	..	Every night.
*P.r.n., Pro re nata	..	..	..	Occasionally as need arises
Qq., Quaque	..	..	..	..	Each or every.
Qq.h., Quaque hora	..	..	..	Each hour.
Qq. q.h., Quaque quarta hora	..	Every four hours.
Q.s., Quantum sufficit	..	..	..	As much as is sufficient.
*S.o.s., Si opus sit	..	..	..	If necessary.
Ss., Semis ..	..	..	..	..	A half.
Stat., Statim	..	..	..	..	Immediately.
Ter.	..	..	..	..	Thrice.
T.d. or t.i.d., Ter die, ter in die	..	Thrice a day.
T.d.s., Ter die sumendum	..	..	To be taken three times a day.

* *P.r.n.* denotes that the drug may be repeated as necessary, the interval usually being stated; a drug ordered *s.o.s.* is given once only.

THERMOMETRIC SCALES

Centigrade Scale

Zero, or $0°C$ = temperature of melting ice at sea level (freezing point).

$100°C$ = temperature of steam given off water boiling under atmospheric pressure at sea level (boiling point).

Fahrenheit Scale

$32°F$ = temperature of melting ice at sea level (freezing point).

$212°F$ = temperature of steam given off water boiling under atmospheric pressure at sea level (boiling point).

Therefore the same interval of temperature is divided into 180 degrees on Fahrenheit scale ($212°-32°$) and 100 degrees on Centigrade scale.

$$\therefore \quad 1°F = \frac{100°}{180} C \text{ or } \frac{5°}{9} C$$

$$\therefore \quad 1°C = \frac{180°}{100} F \text{ or } \frac{9°}{5} F$$

To convert F to C deduct 32, multiply by 5 and divide by 9.
To convert C to F multiply by 9, divide by 5 and add 32.

CENTIGRADE AND FAHRENHEIT EQUIVALENTS

Centigrade: Fahrenheit $F° = (C° × \frac{9}{5}) + 32$				Fahrenheit: Centigrade $C° = (F° - 32) × \frac{5}{9}$					
C°	F°	C°	F°	F°	C°	F°	C°	F°	C°
−50	−58·0	49	120·2	−50	−46·7	99	37·2	157	69·4
−40	−40·0	50	122·0	−40	−40·0	100	37·7	158	70·0
−35	−31·0	51	123·8	−35	−37·2	101	38·3	159	70·5
−30	−22·0	52	125·6	−30	−34·4	102	38·8	160	71·1
−25	−13·0	53	127·4	−25	−31·7	103	39·4	161	71·6
−20	−4·0	54	129·2	−20	−28·9	104	40·0	162	72·2
−15	+5·0	55	131·0	−15	−26·6	105	40·5	163	72·7
−10	14·0	56	132·8	−10	−23·3	106	41·1	164	73·3
−5	23·0	57	134·6	−5	−20·6	107	41·6	165	73·8
0	32·0	58	136·4	0	−17·7	108	42·2	166	74·4
+1	33·8	59	138·2	+1	−17·2	109	42·7	167	75·0
2	35·6	60	140·0	5	−15·0	110	43·3	168	75·5
3	37·4	61	141·8	10	−12·2	111	43·8	169	76·1
4	39·2	62	143·6	15	−9·4	112	44·4	170	76·6
5	41·0	63	145·4	20	−6·6	113	45·0	171	77·2
6	42·8	64	147·2	25	−3·8	114	45·5	172	77·7
7	44·6	65	149·0	30	−1·1	115	46·1	173	78·3
8	46·4	66	150·8	31	−0·5	116	46·6	174	78·8
9	48·2	67	152·6	32	0	117	47·2	175	79·4
10	50·0	68	154·4	33	+0·5	118	47·7	176	80·0
11	51·8	69	156·2	34	1·1	119	48·3	177	80·5
12	53·6	70	158·0	35	1·6	120	48·8	178	81·1
13	55·4	71	159·8	36	2·2	121	49·4	179	81·6
14	57·2	72	161·6	37	2·7	122	50·0	180	82·2
15	59·0	73	163·4	38	3·3	123	50·5	181	82·7
16	60·8	74	165·2	39	3·8	124	51·1	182	83·3
17	62·6	75	167·0	40	4·4	125	51·6	183	83·8
18	64·4	76	168·8	41	5·0	126	52·2	184	84·4
19	66·2	77	170·6	42	5·5	127	52·7	185	85·0
20	68·0	78	172·4	43	6·1	128	53·3	186	85·5
21	69·8	79	174·2	44	6·6	129	53·8	187	86·1
22	71·6	80	176·0	45	7·2	130	54·4	188	86·6
23	73·4	81	177·8	46	7·7	131	55·0	189	87·2
24	75·2	82	179·6	47	8·3	132	55·5	190	87·7
25	77·0	83	181·4	48	8·8	133	56·1	191	88·3
26	78·8	84	183·2	49	9·4	134	56·6	192	88·8
27	80·6	85	185·0	50	10·0	135	57·2	193	89·4
28	82·4	86	186·8	55	12·7	136	57·7	194	90·0
29	84·2	87	188·6	60	15·5	137	58·3	195	90·5
30	86·0	88	190·4	65	18·3	138	58·8	196	91·1
31	87·8	89	192·2	70	21·1	139	59·4	197	91·6
32	89·6	90	194·0	75	23·8	140	60·0	198	92·2
33	91·4	91	195·8	80	26·6	141	60·5	199	92·7
34	93·2	92	197·6	85	29·4	142	61·1	200	93·3
35	95·0	93	199·4	86	30·0	143	61·6	201	93·8
36	96·8	94	201·2	87	30·5	144	62·2	202	94·4
37	98·6	95	203·0	88	31·0	145	62·7	203	95·0
38	100·4	96	204·8	89	31·6	146	63·3	204	95·5
39	102·2	97	206·6	90	32·2	147	63·8	205	96·1
40	104·0	98	208·4	91	32·7	148	64·4	206	96·6
41	105·8	99	210·2	92	33·3	149	65·0	207	97·2
42	107·6	100	212·0	93	33·8	150	65·5	208	97·7
43	109·4	101	213·8	94	34·4	151	66·1	209	98·3
44	111·2	102	215·6	95	35·0	152	66·6	210	98·8
45	113·0	103	217·4	96	35·5	153	67·2	211	99·4
46	114·8	104	219·2	97	36·1	154	67·7	212	100·0
47	116·6	105	221·0	98	36·6	155	68·3	213	100·5
48	118·4	106	222·8	98.6	37·0	156	68·8	214	101·1

11 STERILIZATION: PRINCIPLES AND PRACTICAL APPLICATION

Sterilization in the surgical sense means the process whereby a substance or body is rendered free from living organisms, and under this term are included various methods of killing bacteria and other micro-organisms.

All instruments, utensils and dressings used in the conduct of surgical dressings and other procedures for which aseptic precautions are necessary must be sterile and must then be handled only by a person with surgically clean gloved hands or with sterile forceps.

The word "asepsis" implies the absence of micro-organisms, while "antisepsis" (against sepsis) usually implies the use of chemical disinfectants to kill micro-organisms. Aseptic precautions in a ward or theatre imply that all dressings and appliances are sterile and that there is no risk of contaminating the wound and while similar precautions are taken with septic cases, additional antiseptic precautions may be taken to prevent spread of infection.

It cannot be too strongly emphasized that all dressing utensils and materials must be kept free from contamination with gross dirt even if they are to be sterilized before use. Any method of sterilization will be ineffective unless the equipment is thoroughly cleaned beforehand. Any organic matter, such as blood, pus or excreta, will form a barrier to full penetration by the sterilizing agent. A further point which is not always appreciated is that aseptic precautions are as necessary in dealing with an infected wound as with a clean one. The danger to the patient is increased if a fresh infection is introduced.

Complete sterilization of instruments and equipment used in surgical practice is usually effected by exposure to high temperatures for a sufficient length of time to kill all living organisms and their spores. There are other physical means such as exposure to gamma rays in an atomic pile or irradiation by radioactive cobalt which are already being used and likely to be developed in the near future, and will be particularly useful for sterilizing equipment which is readily damaged by heat, such as rubber articles and some endoscopes. Up to the present time, however, heat is the most generally used, and the most efficient agent, wherever its use is possible, in the form of high-pressure steam sterilizers (autoclaves) and hot-air ovens; boiling-water sterilizers are also still in common use and with proper care and precautions can be regarded as reasonably safe for the sterilization of metal equipment such as instruments and bowls.

Disinfection by chemical agents is an ancillary method for materials and equipment which cannot stand exposure to heat, such as some endoscopes; chemical agents are also used for disinfection of the skin and the irrigation of body cavities.

Sterilization by Physical Means

Heat kills all forms of bacterial life, although those organisms which can take on a protective spore formation can withstand a higher temperature for a longer period than the less resistant, or vegetative, forms.

Autoclaving

Steam kills organisms by coagulation of the cell protein, provided that certain factors are present; the steam must be under pressure, dry and saturated. With these conditions fulfilled, the steam will condense when it meets the cooler surface of the articles in the autoclave and the latent heat released on condensation, will penetrate and kill the organisms. Autoclaving at a pressure of 20 lb. per square inch (above atmospheric pressure) and a temperature of 126°C (260°F) for twenty minutes is an efficient method of sterilizing fabrics such as gowns, towels and dressings, and also instruments. The latest types of high-speed, high-vacuum autoclave operating at higher temperatures reduce the time needed for sterilization. Rubber is readily damaged by exposure to high temperatures for long periods such as are necessitated during the process of creating a vacuum and subsequent drying process in all but modern autoclaves. Rubber gloves are usually autoclaved at a lower temperature, *e.g.* 121°C (250°F), for ten minutes. The gloves should be very loosely packed in order to ensure full penetration of the steam.

It is important to remember that any sterilization by autoclaving is reliable only if the autoclave is correctly installed and efficiently operated, and the materials are packed loosely so that all parts are accessible to the steam. The operation of an autoclave is a serious responsibility and should be entrusted only to one who understands its working. Tests of efficiency, in addition to checking the accuracy of the pressure gauges and temperature readings, should be carried out at regular intervals; these include indicators, control tubes and bacteriological tests.

Boiling

All pathogenic organisms in the vegetative form and many spore forms are killed by five minutes' immersion in boiling water, although there are resistant spores which will withstand long periods of boiling. If the water is made alkaline its lethal effect is increased; therefore sodium carbonate is added to the water in which instruments are boiled, if this method of preparation is used. A 2 per cent. solution of sodium carbonate also retards rusting and reduces the blunting of sharp instruments during boiling. In order that this method of sterilization may be as efficient as possible the following points should be carefully observed:

(1) The water must be boiling for the full five minutes. The addition of a large number of cold metal instruments to the water takes it off the boil. The water must be boiling again before the five minutes' timing is begun.

(2) All instruments in the sterilizer must be completely immersed in the water.

(3) After use all instruments must be boiled for five minutes and carefully dried before being put away.

(4) Instruments when not in use must be stored in a dust-free and dust-proof instrument cupboard.

(5) The material to be sterilized must be either a good conductor of heat, such as metal, or so constructed that all surfaces are easily reached by the boiling water. Material such as thread wound on reels requires a longer period of boiling because the heat does not at once penetrate to the inner layers.

In cases where contamination with spore-forming organisms,

such as anthrax or tetanus organisms, is suspected all instruments and other articles which have been used should either be autoclaved or be subjected to prolonged and repeated boiling. The articles should first be boiled for one hour and after a period allowed for cooling the boiling should be repeated for a further hour. Any spores which have escaped destruction will revert to the vegetative form during the interval and are then killed during the second boiling.

Dry Heat

This kills micro-organisms by oxidation, and provided that the articles to be sterilized are exposed to a temperature of 160°C (320°F) for one hour all organisms and their spores will be destroyed. This method is suitable for all types of glass ware, including glass syringes (but not glass and metal syringes where solder will melt in the high temperature in the oven) and some instruments such as knife blades and skin-grafting knives.

Other Physical Agents

Other physical agents in addition to heat will destroy bacteria, but, with the exception of gamma radiation, have not a very wide practical application in hospital practice.

Cold. Most organisms will survive exposure to very low temperatures but will not multiply. A practical application of this is the preservation of foodstuffs in cold storage.

Light. Direct sunlight kills many bacteria including the tubercle bacillus. The active agent is the ultra-violet radiation and these rays have been used to sterilize milk and water.

Drying. Moisture is as important to most bacterial cells as it is to tissue cells and removal of water will kill the cell. In certain circumstances, however, some bacteria can survive drying for considerable periods and are therefore likely to be present in dust. Examples are pyogenic organisms, diphtheria bacillus and the *Mycobacterium tuberculosis* in pus and sputum.

Gamma Radiation. This agent is being increasingly used for materials which cannot be effectively sterilized by heat without damage. A number of packaged disposable items of surgical equipment, such as plastic catheters, knife holders and tubing; suture materials are also sterilized by this method.

Chemical Disinfectants

It is essential that the nurse should understand the necessary conditions for the effective use of these agents, otherwise chemical disinfection may be quite useless and may even be dangerous if it gives rise to a false sense of security.

(1) To be efficient the disinfectant must be sufficiently strong and must be allowed to act for a sufficient length of time.

(2) With very few exceptions the disinfectant must be in solution; dry powders have very little effect.

(3) The disinfecting power of the agent varies with the number of organisms present; highly infected material is difficult to disinfect efficiently.

(4) The disinfecting power of the agent is to a certain extent dependent upon the nature of the medium containing the organisms, e.g. the germicidal power is lowered in the presence of pus since in this medium many of the organisms are inside the dead leucocytes and it is difficult for the disinfectant to reach them.

(5) As a general rule it may be stated that disinfectant solutions are more effective hot than cold.

(6) Spore-forming bacteria and the acid-fast group (of which the *Mycobacterium tuberculosis* is the most important member) are much more resistant to the action of liquid disinfectants than they are to the action of heat.

(7) Disinfection usually proceeds more rapidly in an acid than in an alkaline medium.

Principal Groups of Chemical Disinfectants

A great many chemical substances are in use as disinfectants or antiseptics, many of them under proprietary names. The terms "bactericide" and "bacteriostatic", the former referring to substances which kill bacteria, and the latter to substances which inhibit bacterial growth, more accurately define the action of certain agents such as antibiotics than the words "disinfectant" and "antiseptic". At the end of this chapter a list of disinfectants, antiseptics and lotions will be found, with some notes on their particular uses.

Oxidizing and Reducing Agents. Hydrogen peroxide in the presence of organic matter readily yields oxygen and in so doing acts as a mechanical cleansing agent removing pus and debris from a wound or cavity.

Potassium permanganate is an oxidizing agent with deodorant properties. Sulphur dioxide and formalin are reducing agents which alter the nature of the bacterial cell by removing oxygen.

Halogens. These substances are a group of non-metallic elements including chlorine, iodine and bromine, the first two, chlorine and iodine, having very wide uses as disinfectants.

The chief chlorine compounds used are eusol, Dakin's solution, chloramine and electrolytic sodium hypochlorite (Milton). These solutions liberate free chlorine which combines with proteins in the tissues and in bacterial cells. The solution has a cleansing as well as a disinfectant action since the protein of necrotic tissue and sloughs is dissolved and washed away. A chlorine derivative of xylenol, chloroxylenol, is known under a variety of proprietary names, e.g. Dettol and Osyl. More recent chlorine compounds are chlorhexidine (Hibitane), benzalconium chloride (Roccal) and hexachlorophane, which is used in antibacterial soaps, such as Cidal, and in a hand-washing cream, Phisohex.

Iodine, like chlorine, has the power of combining with proteins. It is relatively insoluble in water but will dissolve in a solution of potassium iodide. The commonly used preparation "tincture of iodine" (Weak Solution of Iodine, B.P.) is a $2\frac{1}{2}$ per cent. solution with potassium iodine in alcohol.

Salts of Heavy Metals. These substances are first adsorbed on to the surface of the bacteria and then penetrate the organisms and kill them. The bactericidal power of most of these chemicals is, however, reduced in the presence of serum and other organic matter. Water-soluble mercurial salts, in low concentrations, are effective disinfectants for many purposes but they are irritating to the skin, tarnish metals and become relatively inactive in the presence of blood, pus and other organic matter, such as excreta. Perchloride of mercury is one of the oldest of the mercurial disinfectants and is the one in which the disadvantages just mentioned are most marked. Compounds containing very small amounts of mercury, phenylmercuric acetate and phenylmercuric nitrate, are suitable for chemical sterilization of some delicate instruments such as cystoscopes of the non-boilable type. Oxycyanide of mercury is another example of a mercurial disinfectant.

Cresol and Phenol Disinfectants. Carbolic acid is well known as the disinfectant introduced into surgical practice by Lord Lister. It is feebly acid in watery solution, but has a marked caustic action. A 5 per cent. solution will kill all vegetative bacteria and most spores in one hour; a 1 per cent. solution will kill most non-sporing organisms in ten minutes. Tar acid preparations (containing phenol, cresols, etc.) in the form of black disinfectant fluids, such as Cyllin, and white disinfectant fluids, such as Izal and Jeyes fluid, are specially suitable where large quantities of the solution are needed, as, for example, disinfecting excreta, bedpans and linen. Their disadvantages are that they are sticky and there may be some difficulty in rinsing and cleaning utensils afterwards, also the black fluids may stain linen. A proprietary disinfectant, Sudol, contains 50 per cent. phenol and is a useful solution for general disinfection of such items as linen, baths, washing bowls and sanitary utensils. Lysol is a soapy solution of cresol containing 25 per cent. soap. It is more expensive than crude phenol preparations and should be used with economy. All Cresol and phenol preparations are potentially dangerous poisons even in dilute solution.

Chlorine derivatives of cresol and xylenol, chlorocresol and chloroxylenol, are less caustic than carbolic acid or lysol.

Aniline Dyes. The flavine group of dyes is not used very widely now in surgical practice. Acriflavine was the preparation most frequently employed; proflavine is, however, more easily prepared and less irritating to the tissues than acriflavine. The flavine dyes have a specific action on staphylococci and streptococci and their activity is not decreased by the presence of serum. 5-Amino-acridine is a newer addition to the series and is practically non-staining. Other aniline dyes such as brilliant green and gentian violet are sometimes used in the form of skin paints.

Cationic Detergents. These solutions, of which cetrimide and cetavlon are examples, have a detergent action removing grease and with it dirt and bacteria. They are not compatible with soap. Detergents are used for the cleaning of the hands, and of the skin of operation sites and for cleansing wounds. A proprietary preparation, Savlon, is a combination of cetrimide and chlorhexidine.

Another example of a cationic bactericide is domiphen bromide (Bradosol) which can be used for a number of different purposes, *e.g.* disinfection of linen and utensils, hand lotion and mouth wash.

Bactericides and Bacteriostatics which can be Given Internally

One of the most outstanding advances in medical science during the past thirty years has been the development of bacteriostatic and, in some cases, bactericidal preparations which can be given orally or parenterally to combat infection in the living tissues.

One main group of these preparations is known as the chemotherapeutic substances. These include the sulphonamides, such as sulphadimidine, sulphadiazine and sulphamethoxpyradazine (Ledermycin), which are effective against a large number of both Gram positive and Gram negative organisms, sulphone compounds used in the treatment of leprosy, isonicotinic acid hydrazide (INAH) and para-aminosalicylic acid (PAS), both of which are used in the treatment of tuberculous infection.

The second group is known as the antibiotics, so called because they are derived from living organisms, as distinct from inorganic chemical compounds. The first antibiotic to be used in clinical practice, and still the most commonly employed, is penicillin, obtained from the mould *Penicillium notatum*. There are large numbers of penicillin preparations at present available and their number is continually increasing. Examples of these are benzyl penicillin, penicillin G, and methicillin (Celbenin). A substance obtained as a metabolic product of Penicillium moulds, griseofulvin (Fulcin) is used specifically in the treatment of fungal infections, such as ringworm, which are often resistant to local applications. Penicillin is effective in most pyogenic infections but resistant strains of the infecting organism, particularly staphylococci, can be produced and some individuals show a sensitivity to penicillin; usually it is in the form of an urticarial rash but sometimes serious anaphylactic shock occurs. Antibiotics with a similar action to penicillin have been developed for use where the micro-organisms have become resistant, or the patient sensitive, to penicillin. Examples of these are erythromycin and oleandomycin.

The "broad spectrum" antibiotics are so called because they are effective against a number of different types of organisms and are useful in mixed infections. This group includes chloramphenicol (used mainly in the treatment of *Salmonella typhi* infections) and the tetracyclines, such as oxytetracycline, Aureomycin and Terramycin (Ledermycin).

Streptomycin, obtained from *Actinomyces griseus*, was the first effective drug for the treatment of tuberculous infection, and this is still its main role, although it may be given in urinary infections and in countries where bubonic plague occurs it is used in the treatment of this disease. Streptomycin is never given alone in the treatment of tuberculosis, but is combined with INAH or PAS, or both, since it has been found that if a combination of these drugs is used there is less risk of the organisms becoming drug resistant. Other anti-tuberculosis drugs are now available but are usually reserved for cases which have become drug resistant, examples of these are cycloserine and ethionamide.

A third group of antibacterial drugs which are not related either to the sulphonamides or the antibiotics is known as the nitrofurans. Nitrofurazine (Furacin) is used in the treatment of various skin conditions and it is stated that it is effective against *Staphylococcus aureus* infections. Another member of this group, nitrofurantoin (Furadantin) is used in the treatment of genito-urinary infections.

For further information regarding the range and uses of chemotherapeutic and antibiotic drugs the student is referred to appropriate textbooks of medical and surgical treatment.

Cleaning and Sterilization of Instruments, Dressing Equipment and Materials

Instruments

Most metal instruments can be boiled for five minutes in water containing 2 per cent. sodium carbonate. Sharp instruments may also be boiled if they are wrapped so as to prevent contact of the sharp edges with the sides of the sterilizer during the process. Instruments are usually dished dry into sterile trays or boxes covered with a properly fitting lid. Instruments may be sterilized in the autoclave, this is the method increasingly employed in operating theatres and used in central sterile supply departments.

Particularly delicate instruments call for special methods of sterilization and the nurse should ascertain the method to be adopted in each case; some cystoscopes, for example, are boilable and may be placed in the perforated metal box in which they are stored in a sterilizer containing warm water which is brought up to boiling point and allowed to boil for five minutes. The telescope, light and light carrier of non-boilable types of cystoscopes and endoscopes are damaged by boiling and may be sterilized in a formalin cabinet, or in a solution such as 1–10,000 phenyl

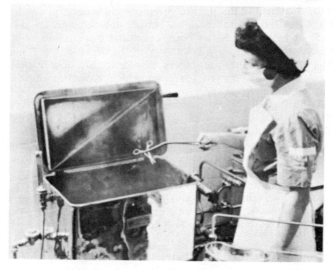

(*Camera Talks*)

Fig. 11.1. When instruments are boiled they must be clean before they are put into the sterilizer, immersed completely in boiling water and left for at least five minutes.

mercuric nitrate or Hibitane 2 per cent. for twenty minutes; valves and irrigating nozzles may be boiled for five minutes.

After use instruments are washed in cold water and then scrubbed in hot soapy water using a brush kept for the purpose. They should then be boiled for five minutes and afterwards dried. Joints and grooves require special care both in cleaning and drying. Stainless steel instruments need no other treatment except periodic oiling of the joints.

Glass Articles

Among glass articles can be included glass connections and funnels.

If these articles cannot be sterilized in a hot air oven they can be boiled, but should not be plunged straight into boiling water. They may be warmed in hot water first, placed in a sterilizer and gradually brought to the boil and boiled for five minutes. To

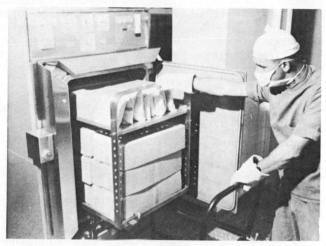

(*Camera Talks*)

Fig. 11.2. Instruments and dressings may be sterilized in an autoclave where they are subjected to steam under pressure according to a pre-determined cycle.

reduce the risk of breakage they should not be with other articles, especially heavy instruments.

After boiling and before use glass articles should be inspected for cracks or chips.

Plastic Instruments and Equipment

Some instruments, especially those for diagnostic purposes, are now made with plastic parts which require special care in sterilization. "Coldlite" auriscopes, diagnostic sets and rectal and vaginal speculæ are examples of these. "Coldlite" instruments of clear plastic with metal attachments can be boiled for five minutes in plain water, but must be wrapped to prevent scratching. These instruments should never be sterilized by immersion in phenol, lysol, or any other acid disinfectant, nor should they be allowed to come into contact with instruments which have been so treated, as any trace of these disinfectants will cloud the transparent plastic. Methylated or surgical spirit will also cause discoloration. These instruments cannot be autoclaved. Cetrimide, 1 per cent. solution may be used, but instruments should not be kept continuously in such a solution and should be washed and dried as quickly as possible after use. The lamps of any illuminated instruments must be removed before boiling; they may be cleaned when necessary by wiping with spirit, but immersion in spirit or any solution will weaken the cement.

Polythene tubing and catheters can also be boiled for five minutes. Some types of plastic material will not stand autoclaving and are sterilized by gamma radiation.

Sterilization of Syringes

Two main types of syringes are in use for the injection of drugs and for the withdrawal of blood or aspiration of pus or fluid. These are the "Record" type, which are partly glass and partly metal, and the all-glass type. Disposable nylon syringes are available. These are supplied ready sterilized with the needle in a packet. They are not suitable for all drugs and for this reason all-glass syringes and disposable needles may be preferred for injection purposes. Syringes should be sterilized by heat. Chemical disinfectants are not recommended for this purpose for several reasons, the action of the chemical is often slow and the disinfectant cannot with certainly be assumed to have penetrated into all the crevices of the syringe; traces of the disinfectant remaining in the syringe may damage or alter the solution to be injected. The rinsing of the syringe after removal from the disinfectant is a possible source of danger, sterile water is readily contaminated once the container is opened; therefore, unless an autoclaved and previously unopened bottle can be provided for each rinsing, there is a possibility of contaminating the syringe and its contents. Drawing alcohol through a syringe before use as a means of sterilization has been demonstrated to be ineffective. Immersion of the syringe in 70 to 75 per cent. alcohol for five minutes is considered safe if the all-glass syringe is used. This method can be used, for example, for a diabetic patient's injection of insulin, provided that the syringe is washed well before the immersion and when it is rinsed after removal from spirit, precautions are taken to ensure that the water used for this purpose is freshly sterilized.

The best method of sterilization for all-glass syringes is by hot air at a temperature of 160°C (320°F) for one hour, this exposure will kill vegetative and spore forms of bacteria. The syringe can be assembled before sterilization and placed in a glass or metal container. Needles are also best sterilized with the syringes in the hot air oven. The containers must be efficiently sealed, and for this purpose thin aluminium foil is suitable. Sterilization may be

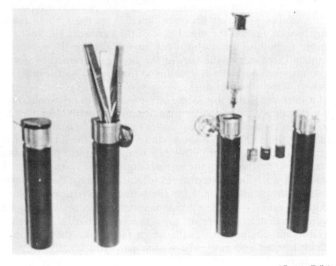

(Camera Talks)

Fig. 11.3. Sterilization by dry heat is useful because instruments remain dry and can be sterilized and stored in sealed containers.

carried out by autoclaving for twenty minutes at a pressure of 20 lb. and a temperature of 120°C but penetration of the steam to all parts of the syringe is doubtful if the syringe is assembled before sterilization, and it is possible that the syringe may not be dry after autoclaving.

Although glass and metal syringes which will stand high temperatures are now available, in some types the cement in the glass-metal seal of the nozzle may melt at high temperatures. Boiling in the ward sterilizer may be used for these syringes but cannot be relied upon to kill spores and is, therefore, not a guarantee that the syringe is in actual fact sterile, but it is stated that accidents due to contamination with spore-forming organisms are rare and the method can be considered reasonably safe. The syringe must be taken apart for sterilization as the rapid expansion of the metal piston when heated will crack the glass barrel if the syringe is assembled before boiling. A piece of old linen should be placed on the tray of the sterilizer and the sterilizer filled to a sufficient level with warm (but not hot) water. The lint protects the points of the needles and also prevents the glass of the syringe from being broken against the metal base of the sterilizer. The water is brought to boiling point and the syringe boiled for five minutes. It is then lifted out in the tray of the sterilizer, drained of water and transferred with sterile instrument forceps to a sterile bowl or box with a well-fitting lid.

If a sterilizer is not available, as for example in home nursing, the syringe may be boiled in a small saucepan with a lid. When the syringe has boiled for five minutes the water can be drained off and the syringe left in the saucepan covered by the lid until it is required. Lint should not in this case be used as it will prevent the syringe from drying when the water is drained off. The addition of soda to the water in the sterilizer is recommended for the sterilization of instruments but not for the boiling of syringes, because residual alkalinity of the syringe may affect the material to be injected. In districts where the tap water is very hard the syringes may become coated with chalk which may make the markings difficult to read and cause the syringe parts to fit badly. In such cases it is advisable to use softened or distilled water in the sterilizer. Syringes with plastic pistons are available and it is stated by the manufacturers that they can be sterilized without damage by boiling, autoclaving or by hot air.

All syringes should be washed after use in warm soapy water, using a bottle brush for the barrel, and then rinsed in clean water before drying. Infected syringes, *i.e.* those used for withdrawal of blood or for aspirating pus, should be washed immediately after use in a solution of cold disinfectant, a suitable one is 2 per cent. lysol, before washing in soapy water. Syringes used for those purposes should be kept separate from those used for injections.

The needle should be left attached and the fluid drawn through the syringe and expelled several times. It is essential that the washing out of the syringe should be done at once and that the disinfectant solution should be cold, otherwise the syringe nozzle or the needle may be clogged.

If several similar syringes are being washed and assembled together it is necessary to see that pistons are fitted to the right barrels, slight differences in individual syringes of the same capacity occur and, for correct fitting, identification numbers may be engraved on both barrel and piston. In order to ensure smooth working of the all-glass syringe the piston may be lightly oiled with liquid paraffin before being assembled. Many hospitals now operate a central syringe service which is under the direction of the hospital pathologist. The cleaning, servicing and sterilization of syringes is carried out by technicians and the wards and departments collect their supplies once or twice daily.

Rubber Articles

These may be boiled in plain water without soda or autoclaved.

Rubber gloves should be examined for punctures before sterilization. They may then be placed in a bag with a small metal weight, so that they remain below the surface of the water, and boiled for five minutes. Filling the gloves with water also acts as a weight.

Gloves are usually sterilized in the autoclave at a pressure of 15 lb. for 10 minutes. After inspection the gloves are powdered, wrapped in gauze with a layer separating each glove, and packed in a drum with a small envelope containing powder. Separate drums may be used for the various sizes of gloves in use, or the package may be marked with the size of the gloves that it contains. After use rubber gloves are well washed on both sides with soap and water. If they have been used for a septic case they should be allowed to soak for one hour in 1–40 lysol solution before washing. They should be rinsed, boiled and then dried on a towel. Before being put away they should be inspected for punctures and powdered on both sides.

Rubber is damaged by contact with dry heat such as from a radiator, by grease and by acids.

Rubber tubing after use should be cleaned with cold water, then with hot soapy water and afterwards rinsed. Care must be taken to flush the inside thoroughly.

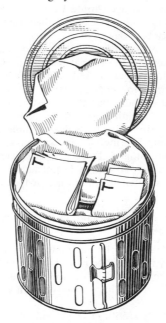

Fig. 11.4. Loosely Packed Drum: Steam Can Reach All Contents.

After boiling, the tubing should be hung over a rail to drain. When put away it should be loosely coiled, avoiding kinking.

Rubber catheters after use should be cleaned by running cold water through from both ends, afterwards washing and rinsing in cold water. They are then boiled for five minutes, dried outside and placed on a towel or hung up until completely dry inside. Stiffened rubber (Tieman's) male catheters are sterilized by the same method as soft rubber.

Elastic Gum

Elastic gum instruments such as catheters and bougies need very careful handling and sterilization because the smooth surface is easily cracked and roughened. If this occurs the catheter must be discarded, as it is likely to damage the delicate lining of the

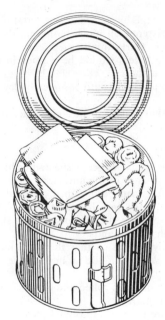

Fig. 11.5. TIGHTLY PACKED DRUM: STEAM CANNOT READILY PENETRATE.

urethra. Bougies and ureteric catheters made of elastic gum may be sterilized by the same methods used for elastic gum catheters.

Two methods of sterilization are:

1. The catheters are wrapped in old linen tied either end with a length of tape or placed in a bag. They are then immersed in boiling water for two minutes, removed by the tapes or bag (not by grasping the catheters with forceps), and placed in a sterile dish or jar containing cold sterile water to stiffen them.

2. The catheters may be placed in a special airtight jar or cabinet containing paraform tablets which evolve formaldehyde gas. Twenty-four hours are required for sterilization by this method. When removed from the jar the catheters should be placed in a dish of sterile water for rinsing, as formaldehyde is irritating.

If a cabinet is available in which the paraform tablets can be heated, the process goes on much more quickly and sterilization may be complete in thirty minutes.

After use the catheters should be washed in the same way as glass and rubber catheters. They should be dried on the outer surface and left on a towel until completely dry before being put away.

It seems likely that plastic, disposable catheters will increasingly replace elastic-gum.

Dressing Materials

Cotton wool, gauze, Gamgee tissue and cellulose are sterilized by steam under pressure in the autoclave.

Dressing materials can be obtained cut ready for sterilization and in a variety of sizes and shapes. If this task is carried out by the nurse in the ward the cutting and packing should be done on a clean towel with clean hands.

Gauze is usually folded so that there are no raw edges. For theatre mops the gauze is made up into squares of different sizes and the edges may be sewn.

Swabs are made of wool rolled and cut into suitable sizes or of wool covered with gauze.

The dressings are made up into packets and put into drums or other containers. Drums are lined with lint or brown paper. Separate packs containing sufficient material for one dressing or procedure may be used. Mass packing of dressing materials in one container involves a risk of contamination and may also encourage wasteful use of dressings. In any event the drum should not be tightly packed as the steam may then not permeate all the contents.

For theatre use it is more usual to pack one type of article in one drum, *e.g.* swabs in one drum, gowns in another, towels in another, and so on. The perforations at the sides or top of the drum are opened just before the drum is put in the autoclave, so that the steam can penetrate. When removed from the autoclave the perforations are immediately closed.

A nylon film has been introduced under the name of "Portex Autoclave Film". This is supplied in a tubular form which can be cut to any desired length and is heat sealed at either end when the articles for sterilization have been packed. The material can be autoclaved as it is permeable to steam, although giving complete protection against external contamination after sterilization.

Disinfectants, Antiseptics and Lotions

Substance	Uses	Strength
Benzalkonium chloride (Roccal).	Disinfection of skin. Disinfection of linen and utensils, also deodorant.	1–10 solution. 1–40 solution.
Chloroxylenol and similar preparations, e.g. Dettol and Osyl.	These preparations are less irritating and less caustic than phenol or cresol. Disinfection of linen and utensils. Antiseptic hand lotion.	1–20 to 1–40 solution. 1–40 to 1–100.
Chlorhexidine (Hibitane).	Skin disinfection. Disinfection of instruments.	1–100 solution or weaker.
Chlorine, in the form of hypochlorite solutions, e.g. eusol, Electroyltic hypochlorite (Milton).	As a dressing or irrigating lotion in the treatment of sloughing or infected tissues. For disinfection and storage of infants' feeding bottles and utensils.	1–80 solution.
Cetrimide (cetyltrimethyl ammonium bromide).	Cleansing the skin. Cleaning utensils.	1–100 solution.
Cresol in soap solution—lysol.	Disinfectant lotion for general purposes. Disinfecting linen and other fabrics.	1–40 solution. 1–80 ($\frac{1}{2}$ oz. to water 2 pints) if linen is left for at least 6 hours.
Domiphen bromide (Bradosol).	Disinfection of utensils and linen. Cleansing wounds and irrigations.	1–500 solution (or weaker).
Flavine group, acriflavine, proflavine, euflavine and 5-aminoacridine.	These dyes are used in the treatment of wounds and as antiseptics on the skin. They may be combined with sterile liquid paraffin as an oily dressing.	1–1,000 solution in water or spirit. (Proflavine is not soluble in spirit.)
Formaldehyde and formalin (a solution of formaldehyde in water).	For disinfecting articles which cannot be treated with steam, e.g. books and leather articles, for fumigation of rooms.	If used as a spray, 8 ounces of formalin to 1 gallon of water for every 400 square feet of surface.
Paraform tablets, these disintegrate slowly liberating formaldehyde.	For the sterilization and storage of elastic gum articles and endoscopes.	
Liquor boracis et formaldehydi.	A solution of formaldehyde with borax and phenol for storing sterile surgical instruments.	

Disinfectants, Antiseptics and Lotions—*cont.*

Substance	Uses	Strength
Hydrogen peroxide.	Used for the irrigation of wounds and cleaning septic mouth conditions. Is non-poisonous and in the presence of organic matter readily liberates oxygen and helps in the separation of sloughs.	Stock solutions contain either 10 or 20 volumes of available oxygen. Diluted with warm water, as required for use, in 2·5, 5 or 10 volumes.
Iodine.	Used for skin preparation, it is more penetrating than most skin paints especially if the skin is dry.	"Weak tincture of iodine," 1–40.
Mercurial preparations: Phenylmercuric nitrate.	Used for sterilizing certain instruments, *e.g.* the telescopes and sheaths of non-boilable cystoscopes; for preserving fluids and suspensions prepared for parenteral injection. For skin preparation. As a vaginal douche for non-specific infections. For mycotic infections.	1–2,000 to 1–10,000 solution. ½ or 1–1,000 in a water soluble ointment base.
Phenol (carbolic acid).	Liquefied phenol, carbolic acid, *Poisonous and corrosive*, if splashed on the skin should be swabbed off at once with methylated or surgical spirit. Disinfecting linen, crockery and sanitary utensils. Disinfecting excreta.	 1–20. 1–10 for one hour.
Crude phenolic disinfectants, *i.e.* "black" and "white" disinfecting fluids, *e.g.* Jeyes fluid, Cyllin, Izal, etc.	Disinfecting excreta. Disinfecting linen, "white" fluids should be used for this purpose as the "black" disinfectants may stain linen. Scrubbing floors, laboratory or sluice room benches, etc. For local pollution of floors, *e.g.* with sputum.	1–10 solution mixed with excreta for two hours. 1–160 solution for 12 hours. 1–160 solution. Swab with 1–5 solution.
Savlon 0·3 per cent. chlorhexidine with 3 per cent. cetrimide.	Washing equipment, *e.g.* dressing trolleys. Skin cleansing.	1–40 solution. 1–20 solution.
Sodium chloride solutions. Normal saline (Physiological Solution of Sodium Chloride B.P.). Hypertonic salt solution.	Used for bathing and irrigating wounds and cavities: for rectal, subcutaneous and intravenous injection. In the treatment of wounds as baths or irrigations.	9–1,000 sodium chloride in water. 1 to 2–10 solution.
Sudol (contains 50 per cent. phenols).	Disinfectant mop for theatre and dressing trolleys. Disinfecting utensils. Soaking linen.	1–120 solution. 1–40 to 1–60 solution. 1–160 solution.

Suggestions for Further Reading

Prevention of Cross Infection in Hospitals. Medical Research
  Council Memorandum No. 11.
Sterilization Practice in Six Hospitals. Nuffield Provincial
  Hospital Trust.
The Planning and Organization of Central Syringe Services.
  Nuffield Provincial Hospital Trust.
Staphylococcal Infections in Hospital. Ministry of Health. H.M.
  Stationery Office.
Aids to Bacteriology for Nurses. Baillière, Tindall and Cox.
Central Sterile Supply Services. Nursing Times.

12 THE CONDUCT OF SURGICAL DRESSINGS

The particular needs of individual cases and the practice of surgeons in different hospitals will naturally necessitate variations in the setting of dressing trolleys and the conduct of dressings. The methods described here are based on the recommendations of the Medical Research Council's Memorandum "The Prevention of 'Hospital' Infection of Wounds." The chief sources of wound infection are bacteria in the air, either present in dust or in infected droplets from the mouths and noses of ward occupants and staff, and bacteria present on hands, dressings, instruments or in lotions. The Memorandum summarizes the principles which should be understood and practised.

(1) During the period that dressings are in progress precautions should be taken to keep the number of bacteria in the air as low as possible. Domestic activities, sweeping and bed-making, should be completed at least one hour before starting dressings. Floors may be oiled to prevent dust from rising during sweeping. Where space is available a treatment room large enough to accommodate a patient in his bed and the necessary equipment will enable such procedures to be carried out with greater safety of the patient and less disturbance of the ward routine than is the case if all procedures have to be carried out at the bedside. Masks are usually worn by all persons concerned in the conduct of surgical dressings. The mask consists of layers of muslin; a piece of cellophane inserted between two muslin layers forms a mask which is impervious, but light in weight. "Disposable" paper masks are also available and are suitable for use over short periods. Masks should be worn only when performing the duties which demand their use, *e.g.* when surgical operations, dressings or treatment are being carried out, when attending on patients particularly susceptible to infection, such as infants, or for the protection of the wearer when attending to patients suffering

from open pulmonary tuberculosis or other infectious diseases. Masks should never be pulled down and left around the wearer's neck but should be removed when the duties requiring them are completed. The cellophane layer is discarded, the muslin mask then placed in a bowl of disinfectant, such as lysol 1–80 and later washed and boiled.

Wards should be closed to all unnecessary traffic unless dressings can be carried out in a treatment room adjacent to the ward.

(2) Hands, whether wet or dry, scrubbed or unscrubbed, are to be regarded in all circumstances as dirty, and should not be allowed to come into contact with wounds or any material directly applied to wounds. If special types of dressings cannot be managed with forceps sterile gloves should be worn.

(3) Wounds should be kept covered except during the actual dressing procedure and the period for which they are then exposed should be the shortest possible. The skin around the wound should be treated with the same care as the wound itself.

(4) It is easier to keep articles sterile if they are dry. Instruments after sterilization should be dished dry into sterile enamel boxes with lids or into covered bowls. Bacteria are more readily washed into a wound from wet hands and from wet instruments than from dry ones.

(5) Precautions must not be relaxed when dealing with wounds that are already infected.

Preparation of the Dressing Trolley

The dressing trolley should be washed with soap and water or a detergent, *e.g.* cetrimide or a disinfectant solution such as Sudol 1 in 120 and dried before being laid. It must be cleaned and relaid for each dressing. Fig. 12.1 shows a trolley set with sterile equipment on the upper shelf and unsterile equipment on the lower shelf.

Sterilized Dressings and Towels

These are packed in drums or other containers, and it is recommended that individual packets should be used in preference to bulk packaging which necessitates the passage of the same container from one dressing to another and its constant reopening. Sterile towels are needed to surround the area of the wound but they are not necessary as trolley covers and they should not be used to cover sterile articles or as temporary dressings since they are very easily displaced.

A mackintosh may be needed to protect the bed, particularly if the wound requires irrigating.

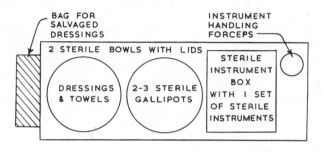

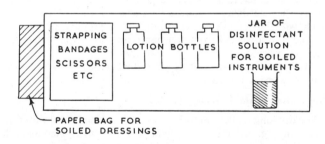

Fig. 12.1. THE LAY-OUT OF A DRESSING TROLLEY.
Top shelf—sterile equipment.
Bottom shelf—unsterile equipment.

Non-Adhesive Dressings

This type of dressing is particularly suitable for raw surfaces and granulating wounds. Carbonet dressings of open-wove gauze, impregnated with water-soluble polyethylene glycol, can be sterilized by autoclaving. Other types of non-adherent dressings, such as Elastoplast "Airstrip" and "N-A" dressings are supplied ready sterilized in individual packs.

Cheatle's Forceps (Instrument handling forceps). These are sterilized by boiling and placed in a tall jar containing lysol 1–40 or other suitable disinfectant solution. The container should be sufficiently deep to keep the blades and the lower half of the handles submerged in the lotion.

Instruments

The instruments commonly needed for ward dressings are dissecting forceps (four pairs should be provided for each dressing), scissors and clip removers. Instruments taken from the sterilizer should be placed in sterile containers with properly fitting lids.

Lotions

Screw-topped bottles of normal saline and water are sterilized by autoclaving before use and care must be taken to prevent contamination of the contents during use. Once open to the air the fluid is no longer sterile unless special precautions are taken. The closed bottle is preferable for irrigating purposes to the open irrigating can, and for this purpose a length of rubber tubing with a clip and a cannula or an irrigating nozzle can be attached to a delivery tube passing through a rubber bung in the neck of the bottle. The whole outfit can be sterilized by autoclaving, or the bottle and its contents may be autoclaved and the fittings sterilized by boiling.

When setting the dressing trolley articles which will be handled by the dresser or the trolley assistant during the actual dressing of the wound are placed on the top shelf, the bottom shelf is reserved for accessories such as bandages. Bins provided with covers are preferable to open "dirty dressings" bowls or receivers and these should be placed on the floor. A jar containing Sudol 1–40 solution, or other suitable disinfectant into which forceps and other instruments can be discarded after use is recommended in place of a kidney dish. Alternatively two paper bags may be attached to the trolley, one for the reception of soiled dressings and one for used instruments.

Since, as has already been stated, hands must always be regarded as contaminated unless covered by sterile gloves, the older method of attempting to sterilize hands by thorough scrubbing has been abandoned in favour of washing the hands in the ordinary way to remove loose particles and surface dirt. The hands are then dried on a clean dry towel. Persons who handle dressing materials and instruments and who carry out the dressing of wounds should endeavour to avoid directly touching any sources of gross contamination, as, for example, soiled dressing material. Sterile material should be handled with forceps. Finger-nails should be kept short and clean. Hands should be kept in good condition by careful drying after washing and by the use of a hand cream, roughness of the skin and cracks are a danger to the dresser and to the patient. Phisohex cream is very suitable for use in wards and departments; it is an effective skin cleansing agent and less irritating to the skin than alkaline soaps.

The Conduct of Dressings

The division of duties between dresser and trolley assistant need to be carefully thought out and understood if good aseptic technique is to be attained. The following rules are based on the Medical Research Council's Memorandum.

Only one wound should be uncovered at a time unless more than one team is working in the ward at once.

Two persons are needed, a dresser who takes off bandages and dressings and attends to the toilet of the wound, and a trolley assistant whose duty it is to look after the trolley and to pass sterile articles to the dresser.

Before commencing dressings both dresser and assistant don masks. These masks need not be sterile but should be boiled and washed after use and placed in a covered receptacle. Sterile gowns and gloves may be needed for some dressings such as burns, which must be regarded as particularly easy to infect. Before the procedure begins the assistant washes and dries her hands.

The dresser turns the bedclothes back gently, removes the bandages and the outer dressing and places these in the bin or in the paper bag provided for this purpose. The dresser then washes and dries her hands. From this stage all work is carried out with sterile forceps, the hands must not come in contact with the wound, the skin around it, sterile dressings lotions or other sterilized material.

The inner dressing is removed with forceps and placed in the destructor bin or in a paper bag.

The assistant opens the sterile dressing packet, taking care to touch only the outside. Any other material required by the dresser is handed to her by the assistant with sterile forceps. The dresser must be careful not to allow her forceps to touch those of the assistant.

The dresser cleans the skin around the wound, changes packing or drains, carries out irrigations or removes stitches as required, using sterile forceps and a strict no-touch technique. Loose particles of skin or stitches that have been removed should be placed on a moistened swab in a large gallipot to avoid the danger of these particles falling into the bed or on to the floor.

The dresser applies the new dressing with forceps and then discards her forceps into the receptacle provided.

The dresser then re-bandages the wound taking care to see that the bandage is correctly and firmly applied so that it will not slip and expose the dressing.

A third helper is useful, if available, to arrange the bed-clothes or hold a limb if necessary. After rendering such assistance the nurse should wash and dry her hands before proceeding to other duties.

At the completion of the dressing the assistant removes the used articles and afterwards washes and dries her hands.

The dresser replaces the bedclothes and then washes her hands.

Dressing Technique using Individual Packs and Instruments Supplied from a Central Sterile Supply Department

The general principles on which the conduct of surgical dressings is based will apply equally in these circumstances; details of technique will vary according to the type of dressing pack used and the method adopted in the individual hospital. As an example, a basic dressing pack may contain the following articles:

(1) A pair of dressing or handling forceps, used first to arrange the equipment when the pack is opened and then to remove the soiled dressings, and after that discarded.

(2) Two pairs of dissecting or dressing forceps for use by the dresser.

(3) One or two disposable metal foil gallipots.

(4) Two paper dressing towels.

(5) Dressing materials, e.g. six wool swabs, four pieces of folded gauze and a square of cotton wool.

Additional instruments, such as sinus forceps, scissors, or clip-removing forceps, are usually sterilized in separate containers.

The dressing pack is placed on the top shelf of a clean dressing trolley and the outer wrapper is removed. The inner wrapper is opened out, holding the corners of the paper; this provides a sterile field on which the instruments and gallipots can be arranged (Fig. 12.2).

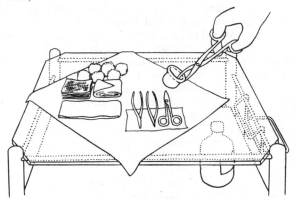

Fig. 12.2. BASIC DRESSING PACK OPENED OUT.
Equipment arranged using handling forceps.

Any extra packs likely to be needed, lotion bottles and the bandage tray are placed on the bottom shelf of the trolley. Two paper bags attached to the frame of the dressing trolley are used as receptacles for soiled dressings and used instruments. When the dressing is completed, the soiled dressings bag is placed in a container provided for this purpose and the bag with used instruments is put in a container for collection by the Central Sterile Supply Department. The bags should be closed by folding the tops over twice.

Removal of Sutures and Clips

For the removal of sutures dissecting forceps and sharp-pointed scissors are required.

When removing interrupted sutures the thread is lifted up with the forceps near the knot and is then cut through between the knot and the skin; gentle traction on the stitch before cutting will expose a portion of the stitch which has been under the skin surface. The thread is then pulled with forceps from the other end towards the incision so that the part that has been lying on the surface is not drawn through the tissues. If a continuous suture has been used it is cut through close to the skin at each point where it has been taken through the tissues. The cut sections are then removed by gentle traction, taking the same care as in the removal of interrupted stitches to avoid drawing the thread that has been lying on the skin surface through the incision.

For the removal of Michel's clips dissecting forceps and clip-removing forceps are required.

The clip is steadied with the dissecting forceps and then one blade of the clip-removing forceps is passed underneath it.

The clip-removing forceps are then closed nipping the clip in the centre, this will bring its pointed ends free of the incision and it can then be lifted out.

Dressing a Wound with a Drainage Tube

Rubber tubing is cut to the required length and one or two holes are made in the side of the tube. A safety-pin is inserted through one end to prevent the tube from slipping into the cavity. The surgeon gives definite instructions regarding the removal of the tube. In some cases it is shortened daily before it is finally removed, this is done by easing the tube partly out of the wound, cutting off the required length and inserting a fresh safety-pin. If a tube is to be taken out during the dressing and later reinserted a duplicate tube, or if ordered, a smaller one, should be sterilized in readiness. If the same tube has to be used again it is cleaned and sterilized before being reintroduced. A rubber drainage tube is inserted by grasping it lengthways with sinus forceps and introducing it in the direction of the sinus track. When dressing the wound a piece of gauze is packed lightly round the tube under the safety-pin. If a tube is not to be removed but it is suspected that discharge has collected at the bottom of the wound a sterile catheter may be passed down the tube and the discharge aspirated with a syringe.

Closed Drainage

Instead of allowing the pus from a cavity to escape via an open tube into a dressing, closed drainage may be employed. This method is particularly useful in draining the pleural cavity, the dressing does not require frequent changing as is the case with open drainage and expansion of the lung is assisted as the tube opens below the level of fluid in the collecting bottle and, therefore, air is prevented from entering the pleural cavity. The drainage tube is provided with a large rubber flange and must accurately fit the incision in the chest wall. It is connected by a

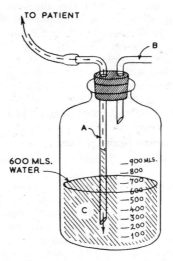

Fig. 12.3. A Drainage Bottle with Underwater Seal.
A. Tube connected to drainage tubing.
B. Air inlet tube.
C. Water seal.

length of tubing to a glass tube passing through the rubber bung of the collecting bottle. The glass tube must be long enough to terminate below the level of the fluid in the bottle. This fluid is usually a measured quantity, *e.g.* 600 ml. of sterile water (Fig. 12.3). When the bottle is disconnected and removed for emptying and cleaning it is important to clip the tubing first, otherwise air will enter the pleural cavity and the partially expanded lung will collapse. It is also important that the tubing shall not be kinked or obstructed and careful arrangement of the pillows and back rest is necessary in order to support the patient without pressure on the tubing (see page 59). A greater degree of suction can be achieved if necessary by attaching an electric pump or a Sprengel's water pump to a short glass connection passing through the bung of the bottle.

13 PREPARATION OF PATIENT FOR OPERATION AND POST-OPERATIVE CARE

Careful pre-operative treatment greatly influences the successful outcome of the operation and the avoidance of post-operative complications. Rest, mental and physical, beforehand is very necessary for the patient who is to undergo a major operation. The nurse's attitude should be one of cheerfulness and confidence but not of indifference to the patient's natural fear and anxiety. The reasons for the various stages of the preparation should be simply explained to the patient before beginning each procedure.

The state of the patient's mouth and teeth should be investigated. The surgeon will decide whether dental treatment is needed. The nurse is responsible for the frequent and thorough cleansing of the patient's mouth as required.

The anæsthetist or the house surgeon will examine the patient's chest. The nurse should report any information that she may have obtained from the patient as, for example, any tendency to bronchitis, a recent cold, an attack of influenza, or the patient's habits with regard to tobacco or alcohol. Breathing exercises may be ordered as a preventive measure against chest complications and these are particularly important in the preparation of the patient for chest and upper abdominal operations.

The bowels should act adequately but violent purgatives tire the intestinal muscle and predispose to post-operative distension. Gentle aperients or enemata are therefore usually ordered, although some surgeons may order castor oil before rectal or perineal operations in order to ensure thorough emptying of the intestinal tract and to inhibit early action of the bowels after operation.

The patient should be encouraged to take sufficient nourishment and the diet should contain a generous allowance of first class protein and vitamins A, B and C. Liberal quantities of fluid and sugar are very valuable, a starved and dehydrated patient is more prone to post-operative complications. If the nature of the patient's disease precludes the intake of sufficient fluid by mouth intravenous administration of saline-glucose solution is likely to be required.

The general cleanliness of the skin should receive attention, the patient having a daily warm bath in bed or in the bathroom.

The nurse's duties include the testing of the urine, the important abnormalities to be looked for are acetone, glucose and protein (albumin).

Consent of the patient or responsible relative for the administration of an anæsthetic and for the operation is required and should be obtained in writing. The patient's blood is usually grouped and cross-matched in case blood transfusion is required.

In the case of women patients coloured nail varnish and lipstick should be removed as artificial colour on the lips and nails may mask cyanosis during anæsthesia.

Safeguards should be taken to obviate the risk of an operation being performed on the wrong patient or on the wrong limb. These include a careful check, usually by the surgeon, to ensure that notes and records are complete and correct and do in fact relate to the patient in question. A label or identification bracelet should be attached to the patient, giving his full name and hospital number. Errors may result if the bed number is used as a means of identification, since beds may be changed round after the admission of the patient.

PRE-OPERATIVE CARE

Preparation of the Skin of the Operation Area

A wide area around the operation site is washed and shaved. The skin is then cleaned with ether, surgical spirit or cetrimide. Some surgeons require no further preparation, others will order the skin to be swabbed with an antiseptic, such as chlorhexidine 0·5 per cent. in spirit. Following this the area may be covered with a sterile dressing and a bandage. The preparation for bone operations may begin three days beforehand although some orthopædic surgeons favour only one preparation. The area is cleaned, repainted and covered with a fresh sterile dressing daily, the last application being made immediately before the patient goes to the theatre. In the case of an emergency operation the preparation of the skin is often carried out in the theatre.

Routine Procedure on the Day of Operation

A hypnotic is often ordered to be given on the preceding evening to promote a good night's rest. If a barbiturate drug is used as pre-medication, *e.g.* Nembutal, the first dose may be given in the evening and the subsequent larger dose about two hours before the operation.

The times at which the various stages of the immediate preparation will be carried out will depend on the time fixed for the operation. The following schedule gives the approximate times when the operation is arranged to take place at 2 p.m. or shortly after.

(1) The early morning specimen of urine is obtained and tested.

(2) A light breakfast of tea and toast is given at 7 a.m. unless there is any contra-indication.

(3) A drink of glucose lemonade or sweetened tea may be given at 10 a.m. unless the anæsthetist's orders are that no fluids should be given after 7 a.m.

(4) At 1 p.m. the patient is dressed in an open-back operation gown. The hair is brushed, a woman's hair if long is plaited, tied and covered with a cap or a triangular bandage. Any jewellery, except a wedding ring, is removed and given into the charge of the ward sister. The patient is given a mouth wash; if he is wearing artificial teeth these are now removed and placed in a porringer.

(5) At 1.45 p.m. the patient empties the bladder or is catheterized if this is ordered.

(6) The hypodermic injection of atropine or other pre-operative medication is given at the time ordered, usually three-quarters of an hour before the patient goes to the theatre.

(7) The patient is placed on the theatre trolley. The form of consent for operation, case notes, X-ray films, a vomit bowl, towel, mouth gag, tongue forceps, swabs and swab-holding forceps are all collected and taken to the theatre with the patient. In a busy surgical ward with long operating lists it is important that there should be a final check of the patient's name, number, notes and X-ray films in order to make sure beyond all doubt that the right patient is being sent to the theatre at the right time.

The nurse accompanies the patient to the anæsthetic room and may remain to assist the anæsthetist, to help wheel the trolley into the theatre and arrange the patient on the operating table. Silence is essential during the induction of the anæsthetic, the nurse should remain quietly at the patient's side and should not speak unless the anæsthetist asks her a question. The ward nurse should be able to answer any questions regarding the patient and his preparation, for example, she should know what pre-medication was given, the time of its administration and the time at which the patient last had any food or fluid.

If a basal anæsthetic such as thiopentone sodium (Pentothal) or pentobarbitone sodium (Nembutal) is given before the patient leaves the ward, he should not be left from the time that the drug is given. Muscular relaxation occurs as the anæsthetic takes effect and the air passage may be obstructed by the tongue falling back. A tray should be ready with a gag, tongue forceps, swab-holding forceps and swabs.

In cases where the operation is a lengthy one, the pre-operative condition of the patient is poor or the loss of blood likely to be considerable, preparations should be made for the transfusion of blood or plasma should this be needed. Oxygen and apparatus for its administration, e.g. a mask or tent, should be ready for immediate use. Oxygen with 5 or 7 per cent. carbon dioxide may be required. Emergency drugs such as nikethamide and nor-adrenaline should be readily available.

POST-OPERATIVE CARE

When the patient is brought back to the ward sufficient helpers must be available to lift him, with the minimum of disturbance, from the trolley to the bed. The head of the trolley should face the foot of the bed. The top bed-clothes are rolled back and if the bed has been warmed, the electric blanket or hot water bottles are removed, and the warmed blanket is placed next to the patient as he lies on the trolley. Three people will be needed to lift an adult patient; all three should stand in a line at the same side of the trolley. One assistant slides her arms under the patient's head and shoulders; the middle helper takes the heaviest weight of the patient's trunk and if a porter assists the nurses this should be his position, the third assistant puts her arms under the patient's legs.

Care should be taken to see that the patient's arm on the far side is not allowed to dangle in such a position that it will be under his body when he is placed in bed. All three persons lift at the same moment, as smoothly as possible, placing the patient gently in the bed.

It is not unusual for a patient to be conscious by the time he returns to his bed in the ward, either because light general, or local, or regional anæsthesia has been used, or because he has been looked after in a recovery unit until the anæsthetist was satisfied with his condition. If conscious the patient is usually placed on his back with one soft pillow under his head. The safest position for an unconscious patient is on his side, so that his tongue falls forward and mucus and saliva can run out of his mouth (Fig. 13.1). In order to prevent him from rolling on to his

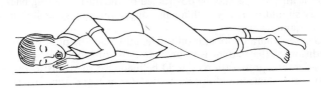

Fig. 13.1. THE LATERAL POSITION.

back the uppermost arm and the uppermost leg are flexed and a pillow can be placed either at his back or against his chest. His head should be in a position of slight extension because this will help to maintain a free air-way.

If the type of operation performed does not permit turning the unconscious patient on to his side, he is placed on his back with no pillow and his head turned to one side. Raising the foot of the bedstead will help to prevent mucus, saliva or vomit from entering the air passages.

The patient must not be left while he is still unconscious, the nurse who remains at the bedside should hold the jaw forward by placing her fingers behind the ascending ramus of the mandible in order to keep the tongue forward and the air-way clear (Fig. 13.2). If an endotracheal tube or a rubber air-way has been left in it should be removed when the patient begins to get restless. The pulse rate should be taken and recorded every quarter-of-an-hour while the patient is unconscious. The strength and volume of the pulse should be noted, also the colour of the patient, the rate and depth of the respirations. If the patient is cyanosed or if his

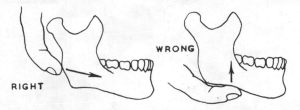

Fig. 13.2. RIGHT AND WRONG WAY OF HOLDING THE JAW OF AN UNCONSCIOUS PATIENT.

respirations are shallow, oxygen may be given after making sure that the air-way is not obstructed.

If the patient vomits his head should be turned well to the side and his mouth mopped out with gauze swabs on sponge forceps. Suction, using an electric suction apparatus or a water suction, is the most efficient method of removing vomit, mucus and saliva from the mouth and pharynx. If his jaw is clenched the gag will be needed and possibly tongue forceps to pull the tongue forward when the mouth is opened. The best pattern of tongue forceps have sharp points which should be inserted into the dorsum of the tongue on either side of the midline and not through the tip.

The dressing covering the wound should be inspected frequently; if any blood or serum soaks through, a sterile dressing should be applied over the bandage without disturbing the original dressing. Any excessive bleeding should be reported at once. Should there be a tube from the operation site that is intended to drain into a receptacle, this must be attended to as soon as the patient is placed in bed, the nurse should also make sure that the tube is not kinked or obstructed in any way. The patient should not be over-heated by too many blankets and may be more comfortable if the operation gown and any extra blankets are removed. If hypothermic ("refrigeration") anæsthesia has been used the patient is placed in an unwarmed bed and covered only by a sheet. The reason for this is to ensure a gradual rise of the body temperature; if the patient is warmed too quickly he may

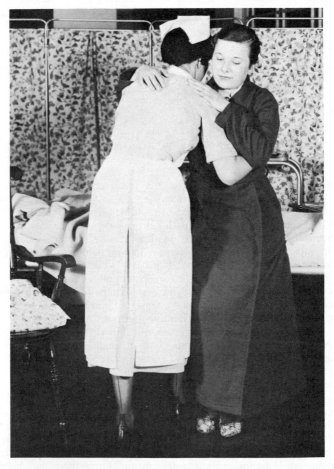

Fig. 13.3. MOVING A PATIENT FROM BED TO CHAIR. I.

This method of supporting a patient from her bed to a chair is used when she is unable to take any weight on the shoulders.

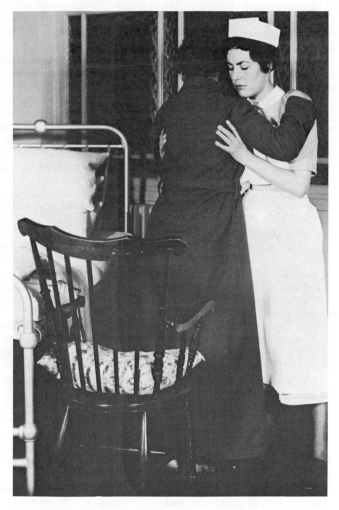

Fig. 13.4. MOVING A PATIENT FROM A BED TO A CHAIR. II.

develop hyperpyrexia. A careful watch on the patient's condition and quarter hourly pulse and blood pressure readings are necessary. Usually, however, these patients are kept in the theatre or the recovery room until the body temperature is normal and the general condition is satisfactory.

Except after operations on the stomach and other special cases in which the surgeon may wish a strict régime to be followed, sips of water may usually be given when the patient has recovered from the anæsthetic. Swabbing the mouth with a pleasant mouth wash will probably be very acceptable to him, and is particularly necessary if he is not allowed to drink. If vomiting occurs, or if for any reason administration of fluids by mouth is not possible, intravenous fluids are usually given.

The measurement of the urine passed should be kept. If the patient has difficulty in passing urine, and is not helped by such simple measures as sitting upright on a bed-pan containing some warm water and the application of warmth over the lower abdomen, an injection of a parasympathetic stimulant such as carbachol, is usually ordered. The patient's bladder must not be allowed to become distended and catheterization may be necessary.

Pain and restlessness should be reported, both will exhaust the patient and may lead to collapse. If morphine or any other sedative has been ordered to be given as and when required, it should be given before the state of exhaustion is reached.

When the patient is fully conscious and his pulse and blood pressure are normal, he is usually nursed in the position which he finds most comfortable. A sitting or semi-sitting position may be favoured as in these positions free movement of the diaphragm is encouraged, with consequent better ventilation of the lungs and less likelihood of accumulation of gas in the intestine. Instances have, however, occurred when patients have fainted in the upright position with very serious results. If this position is used the patient must be carefully watched during the post-operative period. At the first sign or complaint of faintness the pillows should be removed and the patient placed flat in the bed. See also page 59.

The amount of movement which the individual patient can undertake will, of course, depend on his condition and the type of operation. As a general rule the more the patient moves the better, provided that the operation incision is properly supported where necessary. Movements of the foot and ankle joints will help to prevent stiffness and "dropped foot". Exercise of the quadriceps muscles of the thigh will assist the venous return and so help to avoid thrombosis and will also help to maintain muscle tone which is so readily lost with inactivity. Deep breathing exercises will help to prevent stagnation at the bases of the lungs and, by increasing the excursion of the diaphragm, will aid the venous return and also promote peristalsis in the intestine helping to prevent distension and constipation.

After most operations early ambulation is the usual procedure, the patient being assisted from his bed to sit in a chair for a short period within forty-eight hours of the operation. The object of this early movement is to avoid the complications of venous thrombosis and pulmonary embolism. Immobility also favours stasis in the urinary tract with consequent risk of infection and the formation of calculi. The nurse must, however, realize that the fact that the patient leaves his bed does not mean that he is convalescent and he will need a good deal of assistance and encouragement. Everything necessary for his comfort, the chair, blankets and slippers should be prepared and ready before he is moved from his bed and he should be under the observation of the nurse during the whole time that he is out of it.

The time during which the patient will be confined to bed must depend on his general condition and on the nature of the operation. Where firm healing of a plastic operation is essential the patient may be kept in bed for a longer period.

14 USES AND APPLICATION OF BANDAGES

Although a number of methods can be used to secure surgical dressings, there are still occasions when a properly applied bandage is the best way of retaining a dressing in position. Bandages are also used to fix splints, to apply pressure in order to stop bleeding and to give support and prevent swelling, as in the treatment of a sprained ankle.

Types of Bandages

Roller: 4 to 8 yards long, 1 to 6 inches wide. The parts of the bandage are known as the initial end, the drum and the tail.

Triangular: 1 square yard of material cut diagonally makes two bandages.

Many-tailed: Tails 4 inches wide, the length varies from 42 to 72 inches, width of the back 6 to 8 inches. These measurements are for chest and abdominal bandages.

Jaw or four-tailed: 1 yard long, 4 inches wide, before cutting into tails.

T-bandage: for perineal dressings, 1 yard of 4-inch bandage for the waist band, 1 yard of 6-inch bandage for the perineal strap.

Tubular gauze: For limb and head bandages.

Material used for Bandages

Flannel: Strong, warm and gives good support, semi-elastic, but heavy and may be too hot.

Domette: Light in weight, soft and semi-elastic, porous, expensive but washable.

Open-wove cotton: Light and inexpensive, but does not give much support, and the edges fray unless the selvedge edge type is used.

"Kling": open-mesh cotton conforming bandages are very

comfortable, light and porous and are particularly suitable for securing dressings on difficult areas, such as the breast and axilla.

Calico: Harsh and inelastic, but firm; useful for slings and for applying splints.

Crêpe: Comfortable and gives good support, elastic and easy to apply, expensive but washable.

Rules for applying Roller Bandages:

Stand in front of the part to be bandaged.

Pad the axilla or groin when bandaging near these parts.

Start with an oblique turn.

Bandage from below, upwards, and from within outwards.

Applying the bandage with firm even pressure throughout.

Cover two-thirds of the previous turn of the bandage leaving one-third uncovered.

The drum of the bandage must be held uppermost.

Reverse on the outside of the limb.

Finish with a spiral turn, turning in the end of the bandage and securing it with a safety-pin arranged with point uppermost or with a small strip of adhesive tape.

Points to Remember:

The comfort of the patient is the first consideration except when arresting hæmorrhage or correcting deformity.

Two skin surfaces should not be allowed to lie in contact under the bandage; if this point is not attended to, the skin is liable to become moist and sore.

The position of the part—place the limb in the position in which it can most easily be maintained by the patient without strain.

Neatness and economy of bandage should be considered, but the bandage must fulfil its purpose and must always completely cover the dressing.

Various Patterns used in Roller Bandaging:

Spiral: Used for areas of uniform dimensions, *e.g.* fingers.

Reversed spiral: Used for areas of varying dimensions, *e.g.* forearm.

Figure-of-eight: Used chiefly for joints, but can be adapted for use on any part of the body.

Spica: The name given to a figure-of-eight bandage when applied to joints at right angles to the body, *e.g.* shoulder or thumb.

Ear. Use a 2-inch bandage. Fix by placing the end of the bandage over the ear to be bandaged and taking one-and-a-half turns round the head; then carry the bandage obliquely downwards across the back of the head to cover the lowest portion of the dressing. Continue to carry the bandage forwards and upwards across the horizontal turn and over the side of the head. Repeat the horizontal turn. Repeat these two turns until dressing is covered. Finish with a turn round the head and fasten in front.

Eye. Use a 2-inch "fast edge" bandage. Place the bandage over the ear on the side of the eye to be bandaged. Fix by taking a turn

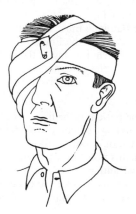

Fig. 14.1. EYE BANDAGE.

across the brow and around the head. Carry the bandage obliquely down across the back of the head, beneath the ear and up over the eye towards the nose and over the head to the starting point (Fig. 14.1). Repeat these turns once or twice and finish by pinning the bandage on the forehead over the good eye. The bandage should not obstruct the vision of the good eye.

Double Eye. First and second turns as for single eye. Third turn carry the bandage down over the uncovered eye, beneath the ear and obliquely up the back of the head. Repeat these turns and finish as before. The crossings should be directly over the nose.

Ascending Spica of Shoulder. Use a 3-inch bandage. Pad the axilla. Fix the bandage with an oblique turn around the arm. Carry the bandage across the back, under the opposite arm and across the chest to the outer side of the arm. Repeat these turns, working up over the shoulder, chest and back until the dressing is covered. Finish over the shoulder in front (Fig. 14.2).

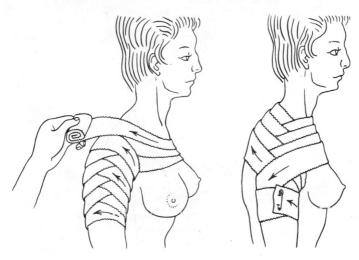

Fig. 14.2. ASCENDING SHOULDER SPICA.

Fig. 14.3. DESCENDING SHOULDER SPICA.

Descending Spica of Shoulder. The same turns are made for a descending spica of shoulder as for an ascending one, but the bandage is begun by placing the end on the shoulder and the spicas work downwards over the shoulder, back and chest. The bandage is finished off by taking a circular turn round the arm (Fig. 14.3).

Breast. (a) *For support or to secure a dressing over a breast abscess.* Use a 4- or 6-inch bandage. Start beneath the unaffected breast and take one-and-a-half circular turns round the body. The bandage is now beneath the affected breast. Carry the bandage obliquely upwards covering the lowest portion of the dressing, over the shoulder and down the back. Repeat the turn round the body, covering only two-thirds of the previous turn (Fig. 14.4). Repeat these turns until the breast is sufficiently covered and supported. Finish in front.

(b) *To secure the dressing following the operation of radical mastectomy.* Use a 6-inch bandage; "Kling" conforming cotton

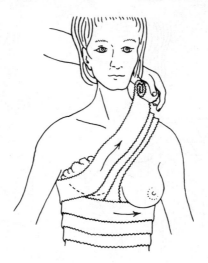

Fig. 14.4. BREAST BANDAGE.

bandages are very suitable for this purpose. Begin by fixing the bandage with a turn around the trunk starting from the side of the operation. Take 2 or 3 spiral turns round the body. Then take spica turns round the shoulder alternating with spiral turns around the trunk until the dressing on the chest and axilla is completely covered.

For all bandages involving the thorax it is important to see that the patient's shoulders are well back when the bandage is applied, otherwise breathing may be impeded.

Flexed Elbow. Use a 2½- or 3-inch bandage. Carry the bandage twice round the centre of the joint. Continue with a figure-of-eight pattern, first above and then below the joint, and covering two-thirds of the previous turn. Finish with a circular turn above the joint (Fig. 14.5).

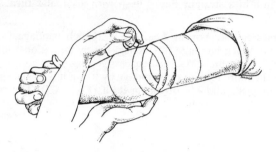

Fig. 14.5. FLEXED ELBOW, DIVERGENT SPICA.

Flexed Knee. Use a 3-inch bandage. The method is the same as for a flexed elbow.

Heel. Use a 2-inch bandage. The same pattern of bandage as for an elbow but the first turn of the figure-of-eight is made below the tip of the heel instead of above. Finish around the ankle.

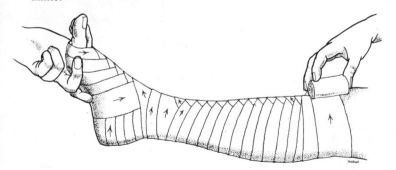

Fig. 14.6. BANDAGE FOR FOOT AND LEG, USING FIGURE-OF-EIGHT AND REVERSED TURNS.

Figure-of-Eight of Arm or Leg. Use a 2- or 2½-inch bandage for the arm and a 3-inch bandage for the leg. Fix by taking one oblique turn round the limb. The pattern is made by carrying the bandage obliquely up, around and down the limb, the loops forming a figure-of-eight. The crossings should be on the outside of the limb in a straight line. Finish with a circular turn. (Fig. 14.6.)

Reversed Spiral, Arm or Leg. Use a 2½-inch bandage for the arm and a 3-inch bandage for the leg. Fix by taking one oblique turn around the limb. As each successive turn is brought to the front of the limb, reverse the bandage by fixing it with the thumb and turning it obliquely down on itself (Fig. 14.7). The points

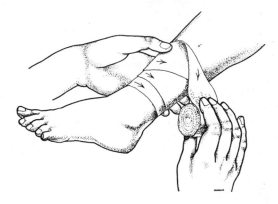

Fig. 14.7. Reversed Turn.

formed in this way should be in a straight line on the outside of the limb. Finish with a circular turn.

Hand. Use a 2-inch bandage. Commence by placing the end of the bandage on the inner side of the wrist, then carry the bandage across the back of the hand to the base of the little finger and take a simple spiral turn one-and-a-half times round the knuckles; the bandage is now by the first finger. Start the figure-of-eight turns round the hand and wrist—three or four should be sufficient. Finish with a circular turn round the wrist. The spicas should come in the centre of the back of the hand. If limited movement of the fingers is not allowed a single layer of material should be placed between them.

Fingers. Use a 1-inch bandage. Start on the inner side of the wrist, leaving a free end for tying. Carry the bandage across the back of the hand to the base of the finger to be bandaged; in one elongated turn bring the bandage to the base of the nail and work down the finger in spiral turns. Carry the bandage across the back of the hand and take one turn around the wrist, and either fasten off by tying the ends together or, if another finger is to be bandaged bring the bandage up the finger and repeat these turns. If bandaging all the fingers, start with the little finger.

To cover the tip of the finger: commence as before, but instead of taking a spiral turn up the finger, carry the bandage straight up the outside of the finger over the tip and down the inside of the finger as far as the second joint; hold the bandage there and make a return loop over the tip of the finger once more. Fix the loops with one circular turn, then, commencing at the top of the finger cover in the whole of the finger with spiral turns as before.

"Tubegauz" is neater and more comfortable than roller bandages for fingers.

Spica for Thumb. Use a 1-inch bandage. Commence from the inner side of the wrist, leaving sufficient to tie. Carry the bandage down between the finger and thumb, then take a single spiral turn around the thumb, followed by a circular turn at the base of the nail. Start the figure-of-eight turns by carrying the bandage across the back of the thumb and hand to the wrist, around the wrist and across the ball of the thumb. Repeat these figure-of-eight turns until the thumb is covered (Fig. 14.8). Finish round the wrist.

Stump. Use a 3- or 4-inch bandage according to the size of the stump. Start by placing the end of the bandage in the centre of the upper side of the stump, then carry the bandage over the centre to the same position on the under side; hold in position with the fingers. Continue to carry the bandage to and fro over the end of the stump until it is completely covered; fix the loops with a circular turn round the stump. Continue up the stump with spica turns until the dressing is covered. The spica of the bandage should be on the upper side of the stump. A crêpe bandage may be used to exert pressure and prevent œdema. Firm bandaging will also help to produce the conical shape of the stump ready for the fitting of the artificial limb.

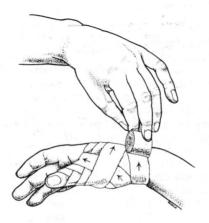

Fig. 14.8. SPICA FOR THUMB.

Ascending Spica of Hip. Use a 4- or 6-inch bandage. Pad the groin. Fix the bandage with one oblique turn around the thigh. Carry the bandage obliquely upwards to the outside of the hip, around the back and down across the pelvis to the outside of the thigh. Continue these two turns, the spica ascending on the front and outside of the thigh. Finish on the trunk in front.

Descending Spica of Hip. Apply in the same way as an ascending spica, but start with a figure-of-eight turn around the trunk and thigh. The spica works downwards instead of upwards and the bandage is finished with a circular turn round the thigh.

Ankle. Use a 2-inch bandage. Start with an oblique turn round the instep and proceed with figure-of-eight turns around the instep and ankle, working upwards with the spica on the front of the foot and ankle until sufficient support is obtained. Finish with a circular turn around the ankle.

The "Barrel" Bandage for supporting a Fractured Jaw. A strip of bandage about 4 feet long and 2 inches wide is required.

This is placed under the chin and tied in a single knot on the top of the head (Fig. 14.9 A). The knot is then loosened and spread out so that one loop passes round the back of the head and the other round the forehead (Fig. 14.9 B). The tails of the bandage are then tied on the top of the head (Fig. 14.9 C).

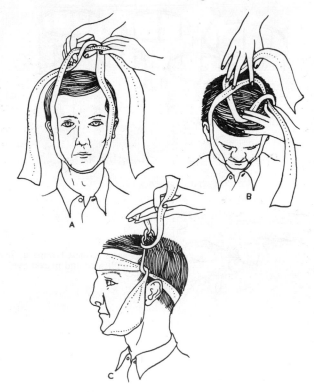

Fig. 14.9. The Barrel Bandage.

"Tubegauz" Bandages

Tubular gauze bandages have recently found favour as a comfortable, neat and efficient method of retaining dressings in position. The gauze is made in various dimensions suitable for many purposes. For bandaging limbs wire cage applicators on which the gauze is stretched are used. (Fig. 14.10.) The applicator is passed over the part to be bandaged and then withdrawn leaving

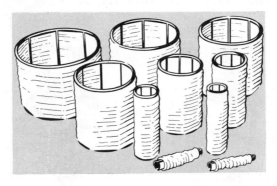

A. Tubegauz Applicators.

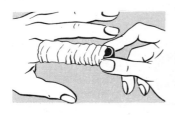

B. Tubegauz gathered onto a finger size applicator and placed over the finger.

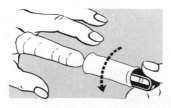

C. Applicator withdrawn and twisted at top of finger.

Fig. 14.10. TUBEGAUZ BANDAGES.

a layer of gauze covering the area. This procedure is repeated to give as many layers as are necessary covering the part.

It is claimed that a great degree of control over the tension of the bandage is possible with this method and also that the bandage will retain its position better than the usual roller bandage. Many casualty departments find that "Tubegauz" is particularly useful for finger dressings and that the light, neat bandage is greatly appreciated by patients. "Tubegauz" also makes a satisfactory and comfortable head bandage.

Triangular Bandages

Triangular calico bandages are used as slings and as First Aid bandages. They are also useful for holding dressings in position on areas where roller bandages would be difficult to apply or would be heavy and cumbrous.

Large Arm Sling (used to support the forearm). Stand in front of the patient. Spread the bandage over the chest, with one end going over the shoulder on the uninjured side, and the other hanging over the abdomen; the point should be beneath the elbow. Place the forearm slightly raised over the middle of the sling; bring the lower end up and tie on the injured shoulder to the other end with a reef knot. Tuck in the ends. Bring the point round to the front of the elbow, fold in neatly and pin (Fig. 14.11 A).

Narrow Arm Sling (used to support the wrist). Make a broad fold bandage by bringing the point to the base and folding in two. Place one end over the shoulder on uninjured side. Place the wrist on the centre of the broad fold and bring the lower end up to the injured shoulder. Join ends with a reef knot (Fig. 14.11 B).

St. John Sling (used when the shoulder is injured and to give support to a fractured clavicle). Place the injured arm across the chest so that the fingers almost touch the opposite shoulder. Place one end of the bandage on the uninjured shoulder so that the point comes well beyond the elbow. Tuck the upper half of the base of the bandage well beneath the forearm and elbow. Carry the lower end across the back and tie the ends on the uninjured shoulder. Tuck the point in between the forearm and the sling. Carry the fold thus made around the outside of the arm and pin firmly to the bandage going up the back (Fig. 14.11 C).

Clove Hitch. To make a clove hitch take a long strip of bandage and with the right hand make a loop, passing the bandage over and then behind the bandage held in the left hand. Make a second loop on top of the first one then slip the top loop behind the first one. (Fig. 14.11 D.)

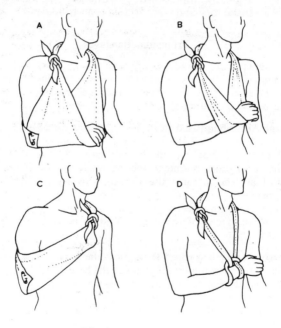

Fig. 14.11. ARM SLINGS.

A, large arm sling; B, narrow arm sling; C, St. John sling;
D, clove-hitched sling.

Scalp. Fold a hem of about 1½ inches along the base of the bandage. Stand behind the patient. Place the bandage over the head with the centre of the base on the forehead, the hem outwards and the point resting on the nape of the neck. Bring the ends around the head, crossing at the back and tying over the centre of the forehead. Draw the point of the bandage down as far as possible, then turn it up and pin it to the bandage on top of the head.

Forehead, Eye and Side of Head. Make a narrow fold by bringing the point to the base and folding in three. Place the centre of the bandage over the dressing, carry the ends around the head and tie.

Chest. Place the centre of the bandage on the dressing, with the point over the shoulder on the injured side. Carry the ends around

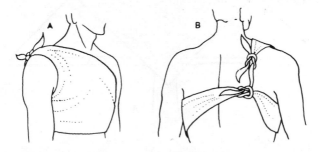

Fig. 14.12. TRIANGULAR BANDAGE FOR THE CHEST.
A, front view; B, bandage secured at the back.

the waist, leaving one end longer than the other. Draw the point over the shoulder and tie to this end (Fig. 14.12).

Back. The back is bandaged in the same way, beginning at the back and knotting the bandage in front.

Shoulder. Two bandages are required. Fold a hem at the base of one bandage and place the centre of the bandage on the shoulder with the point running up the side of the neck. Carry the ends around the middle of the arm and tie on the outer side. Place the arm on the injured side in a broad fold sling, tying the knot over the point of the bandage. Draw down the point over the knot and pin.

Elbow. Fold a hem along the base of the bandage. Place the point of the bandage on the back of the arm and the middle of the base on the back of the forearm. Cross the ends over the middle of the elbow in front and tie around the arm. Bring the point over the knot and pin.

Knee. The same bandage may be applied to the knee.

Hand. Fold a hem along the base of the bandage. Place the wrist on the centre of the base, palm downwards and fingers towards the point. Bring the point over the hand to the wrist,

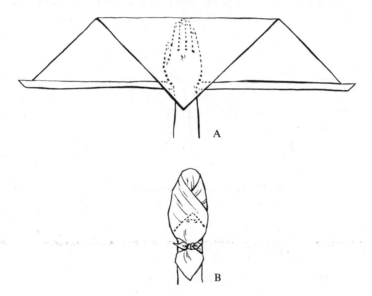

Fig. 14.13. TRIANGULAR BANDAGE FOR THE HAND.
A, first stage; B, completed.

pass the ends around the wrist, or cross and tie. Pull the point over the knot and pin to bandage (Fig. 14.13).

Hip. Two bandages are required. Tie a narrow fold bandage around the body just above the iliac crests, with the knot on the injured side. Pass the point of the second bandage underneath the knot of the first and fold over. Make a hem along the base of the bandage, pass ends round the thigh and tie. Fasten the point of the bandage down with a safety pin (Fig. 14.14).

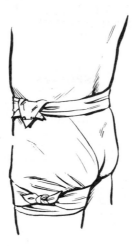

Fig. 14.14. TRIANGULAR BANDAGE FOR THE HIP.

Foot. Place the foot on the centre of the bandage, toes towards the point. Bring the point over the instep. Cross the ends over the instep, carry round the ankle and tie. Pull the point over the knot and pin it.

15 USES AND APPLICATION OF SPLINTS, PLASTER OF PARIS AND TRACTION

SPLINTS

Splints are used to immobilize an injured limb, as in the treatment of fractures, or to prevent movement which might interfere with treatment (for example the use of a straight wooden splint to steady an arm or leg during intravenous therapy) and to prevent or to correct deformities. Examples of these two latter uses are splints used to prevent wrist drop or foot drop where muscles are weak or paralysed and splints used to correct talipes ("club foot") in infants.

The commonest form of splinting in general use is the plaster of Paris splint made for the individual patient. Other types of individual splints made of a variety of materials, such as plastics, resins, leather and metal, are mainly used in orthopædic practice. Some "ready made" wooden and metal splints are, however, still used for a number of purposes; examples of these are:

(1) Thomas's knee splint (Fig. 15.1) used in conjunction with traction in the treatment of fractures of the shaft of the femur.

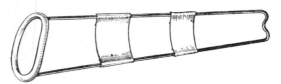

Fig. 15.1. THOMAS'S SPLINT.

(2) Wooden back splint with foot and side pieces, which may be used as a temporary measure in the treatment of fracture near the ankle joint until the swelling subsides.

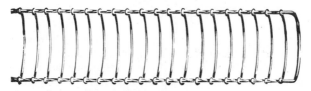

Fig. 15.2. CRAMER'S WIRE SPLINT.

(3) Cramer's wire splint (Fig. 15.2) which can be cut to any length and bent to the required shape.

(4) A metal cock-up splint (Fig. 15.3) used to maintain flexion at the wrist joint.

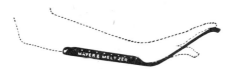

Fig. 15.3. METAL COCK-UP SPLINT.

Padded Splints

In cases where a padded splint is to be applied only as a temporary measure it may be padded with non-absorbent wool fixed by a bandage. When the splint is likely to be needed for some time, a more satisfactory padding is applied as described below.

Requirements:
Calico.
Wool.
Good quality tow, hair is sometimes used for special splints.
Linen thread.
Scissors.
Sewing cotton and needles.

Method. Cut a piece of calico three times the width of the splint to be padded and at least 6 inches longer.

Cut a piece of wool slightly wider and longer than the splint.

Tease sufficient tow to make a thick springy pad, placing the tow on the wool.

Cover the pad with calico, stitch the pad along its length, but leave the ends open.

Place the pad on the side of the splint which will be next to the patient, with the seam of the pad against the splint.

With the linen thread attach the pad to the splint, taking stitches backwards and forwards across the back of the splint, pulling the thread as tightly as possible. Begin 3 inches from the end and finish off 3 inches from the other end.

At each end make a bar by taking several horizontal stitches across the back of the splint.

Turn in the open ends of the calico and attach them to the cross bars at either end with the splint stitch.

Buttonhole stitch along the cross bar to keep the stitches in place.

Application of a Padded Splint, e.g. a wooden back splint and foot piece for the leg.

Requirements:
(1) A padded wooden back splint with foot and side pieces; pieces of dressmaker's wadding or non-absorbent wool are to give additional padding where needed, *i.e.* at the upper margin of the splint, under the upper end of the tibia, or above the heel and over the malleoli.
(2) Two padded side pieces.
(3) An extra roll of wool or wadding.
(4) Webbing straps with buckles.
(5) Dusting powder and wool swabs.
(6) Calico or domette bandages, adhesive strapping.
(7) and (8) Sandbags and a roller towel, or a length of calico 18 inches wide, which may be needed to keep the splinted limb steady.

A large bed cradle is required in order to take the weight of the bed clothes. The leg may first be washed, and if necessary shaved, and lightly dusted with powder. An assistant holds and steadies the limb while the back splint is placed in position, the heel must be right at the end of back splint so that the foot is supported at a right angle by the foot pieces. Extra pieces of padding are put where required and the side splints are applied. The splints are first secured by webbing straps or adhesive strapping and then by firm bandaging. Webbing straps with buckles are useful if the splint is to be removed at intervals for inspection or for exercise of the leg. The splinted limb is supported on a firm pillow; the sandbags and cloth may be used to keep it steady.

Straps, or strapping and bandages, must be sufficiently firmly applied to retain the splint in the correct position, but whenever a splint is applied to a limb the danger of interference with the circulation must be kept in mind. When the bandages are applied, the toes (or fingers in the case of an arm splint) must be left exposed so that their colour can be seen and the circulation tested. Pressure with the fingers over the nails produces blanching; if the colour does not return when the pressure is removed this is a sign of impaired circulation, which must be reported at once. In the meantime the bandages may be cut and the straps loosened without moving the limb from the splint. Frequent tests of the circulation are particularly necessary where there is swelling of the limb. The splint should be comfortable for the patient if it is well padded and properly applied. If there is any complaint of pain over a bony prominence this must receive prompt attention, as unless the pressure is relieved a sore will result.

Plaster of Paris Splints

Plaster of Paris splints are in general use for many purposes. Since the splint is made individually for each patient, it is more efficient and more comfortable than most wooden or metal ones.

The following requirements are usually sufficient for the making of the plaster splint although there may be additions to this list for special plasters:

Pails filled with tepid water for soaking the bandages.

Mackintoshes.

Gypsona plaster bandages of the required widths.

Plaster knives.

Ordinary round-ended scissors and plaster scissors such as Böhler's scissors.

Plaster saw.

Plaster shears will be needed if a plaster has to be removed before the application of a fresh one.

Tape measure.

Blue pencil.

Dusting powder may be used for the patient's skin or, if the plaster is being applied without any padding, the skin may be oiled with olive oil.

A light coating of petroleum jelly may be applied to the inside surface of pails in which bandages are soaked in order to facilitate the subsequent removal of hardened plaster. This is not necessary if plastic pails are used.

A suitable table top or a board is needed for the making of plaster slabs.

Tubular stockinet may be used to cover the limb under the plaster or, in the case of the trunk, a stockinet vest.

Dressmaker's wadding, thick felt or sorbo rubber may be used as padding over bony prominences.

Rolls of "orthopædic" or tailor's wool.

Crêpe bandages.

Open wove cotton bandages.

In the theatre the surgeon is usually already dressed in gloves, a rubber apron and theatre boots; otherwise these should be provided. Canvas over-boots may be used in place of rubber ones.

The pail or bowl provided for soaking the bandages should be deep enough to contain sufficient water completely to submerge the bandages. The bandages are placed in water one at a time and left until all the air has bubbled out of the bandage and the water has soaked through to the centre. When the bubbling has ceased the bandage is removed from the water holding it by both ends and gently squeezed towards the centre so that surplus water is removed but the plaster is not squeezed out.

Plaster Bandages. If Gypsona bandages are not available plaster bandages may be prepared by the following method.

For the foundation of the bandages either butter muslin, which is a thin soft material, or book muslin, which is also thin but stiff, is used. The material is torn into lengths of from one to six yards and varying widths of which four, six and seven inches are the most generally useful. Narrow bandages of one or two inches are usually made one or two yards in length, the wider bandages, six, seven or eight inches, are made in lengths of five or six yards.

The strips of material are folded and loose threads removed. The dry plaster is then rubbed into the material as evenly as possible, using the flat part of the palm of the hand. A short strip of muslin is unfolded at a time and loosely rolled as the plaster is rubbed into the mesh. It is convenient to run a red thread through the free end of the finished bandage so that the end may be easily found after the bandage has been soaked. Until sufficient experience has been gained in rolling plaster bandages some difficulty may be found in gauging the right amount of dry plaster to impregnate the muslin properly so that it is not, on the one hand, so full of plaster that the centre of the bandage remains dry when it is immersed in water and, on the other hand, so deficient in plaster as to be finally little more than a piece of wet muslin. Another common mistake is to roll the bandages so tightly that the water cannot soak completely through and a considerable portion of the bandage is wasted. A fine quality quick-setting plaster should be used. If it has not been stored in airtight tins it may be lumpy, and in this case should be sieved before use. The finished bandages should also be stored in airtight tins and may with advantage be dried out in a warm oven before being put away.

Application of a Plaster Splint

The nurse will often have to assist in the application of the splint, and in some circumstances may be entrusted with the carrying out of the entire procedure. Plaster bandages should be applied evenly but not tightly and no reverses should be made. The bandages should be folded to bring about a change in the direction of the turn. Plaster sets quickly and the moulding of the casting to the limb should be done during the application of the bandages. "Moulding" means pressing the plaster into the natural hollow contours of the part to which it is applied so that it fits the part accurately and pressure on bony prominences is as far as possible avoided. Reinforcement of the splint may be carried out by strips of plaster bandage applied up and down the length of the limb and secured by further circular turns. Metal strips or pieces of Cramer's wire splinting are sometimes incorporated in a plaster splint. The finished splint should not be subjected to pressure, as for example by letting the heel of a leg plaster rest on the table, until it has set; this usually takes about five minutes. The limb should be supported on the flat of the hand in order to avoid making indentations in the plaster. Thorough drying of the plaster takes several hours, the time depending on the size and thickness of the plaster.

Plaster slabs are often used for limbs and have the advantages of being quick and simple to make, supplying a well-fitting splint which can be removed for any necessary treatment. The length is marked on a board or table and wet plaster bandages are folded lengthways up and down the marked area on the board until the requisite thickness is obtained. The slab of bandage is applied to the limb, moulded and then removed and trimmed. The splint is kept in place by a roller bandage.

Plaster shells may be used in the treatment of disease or injury of the spine. These are made by immersing long strips of muslin eight folds thick in thin plaster cream. The strips are applied and moulded on the patient's body usually directly on to the skin which may be previously oiled. One pound of dry plaster mixed with one pint of water makes a cream of the right consistency. The shell is removed for drying, trimmed and lined with wool or Gamgee tissue before use.

Following the application of a plaster the limb should be elevated and the bedclothes arranged over a cradle so as to allow free circulation of air to dry the plaster. The extremities should be inspected hourly for signs of interference with the circulation. If sufficient pressure is applied to a nail to blanch it the colour should return in a few seconds when the pressure is removed. If it remains white for any appreciable time this indicates inadequate circulation; blueness and coldness of the extremities are also danger signs. These signs should be reported at once as the plaster will probably have to be cut away or split and opened. After forty-eight hours, routine morning and evening inspection is in most cases sufficient. A sore may develop under the plaster and any complaint of pain at a definite point or a burning sensation should be reported at once, the area subjected to pressure soon becomes anæsthetic and the fact that the pain has disappeared does not mean that the danger of a pressure sore has passed. If a sore forms, the site may be indicated by the presence of a discharge on the surface of the plaster, the presence of a sore may also be detected by the unpleasant smell which develops when discharge is pent up under the splint. When a leg plaster is carried up to the groin special care is needed to prevent soiling. A piece of jaconet or plastic material may be required for protection of the plaster when the patient uses a bed-pan.

To Remove a Plaster

The plaster should be removed in a plaster room or a ward annexe otherwise infected loose particles are liable to be scattered and will add to the bacterial content of the air in the ward. The plaster should be moistened during the removal to reduce scattering of dry plaster.

A small light plaster can usually be removed by cutting through it with a knife. Great care must be taken to avoid cutting the patient's skin when removing an unpadded plaster, and in this case a pair of plaster scissors is to be preferred. Plaster shears or an electric saw will be required for cutting through a thick plaster.

After removal the plaster cast should be placed in a covered bin. The knives, scissors and shears should be boiled after use.

Plastic Splints

Light-weight splints made of plastics or resins are useful for infants and in cases where the splint is worn for a considerable time as, for example, in the treatment of a fracture of the scaphoid bone in the wrist.

THE APPLICATION OF TRACTION

Traction or extension is applied to a limb in order to exert a steady pull. This may be needed to prevent overriding of the fragments of a fracture or to prevent pain and contractures in the treatment of joint conditions, such as rheumatoid arthritis or tuberculous joints.

Traction may be carried out by the continuous pull of weights, or by fixed traction when the pull is maintained by fixation to the end of the splint. The traction may be applied to the skin of the limb, skin traction, or to the bone, skeletal traction. The latter is obtained by a pin or wire inserted through the bone below the fracture. In the case of a fracture of the lower limb skeletal traction is usually applied at one of three sites, the lower end of the femur just above the condyles, the tubercle of the tibia or the os calcis. For skin traction strips of adhesive material, such as Elastoplast extension strapping, are applied to the skin of the limb, or strips of gauze may be stuck to the skin with Sinclair's glue or Mastisol.

Preparation for Application of Traction

The Bed (see also p. 60):

Fracture boards will be needed to prevent sagging of the mattress.

Blocks are often required for raising the foot of the bed.

A Balkan beam, Hoskin's overhead beam or some other type frame with pulleys, will be needed unless a Braun's frame which forms a cradle and carries the pulleys is used.

The Splint. If a Thomas's splint is used it must be the right size for the patient, the ring should fit comfortably in the groin resting against the ischial tuberosity at the back and the splint should be long enough to project about six to eight inches beyond the sole of the foot. A flexion bar is usually attached to the splint to allow flexion of the knee joint.

Braun's frame is used in the Böhler method of treating fractures of the lower limb. High blocks are required for the foot of the bed and the splint needs to be firmly lashed to the foot of the bed (Fig. 15.6).

Whichever type of splint is used, flannel slings will be needed to support the limb. The slings are double fold, the free ends being fastened to the outer bar of the splint by large "bull-dog" spring clips. When the splint has been applied to the limb each sling is adjusted separately and secured. The upper and lower edges of each sling should overlap the slings above and below, if a gap is left the edges of the sling may press into the soft tissues of the limb.

Support for the foot in order to maintain it in a position of dorsiflexion may be applied in several ways, *e.g.* a foot support attached to the splint, or a cord and a weight attached to a wooden spreader fixed to the sole of a slipper worn on the foot of the fractured limb, the pull of the weight will be towards the head.

The slings should be sufficiently taut to support the limb in a position in which two-thirds of the limb is visible above the level of the metal side bars.

Skin Traction
Requirements:

Adhesive strapping, "orthopædic" strapping, is the most suitable type as it will not stretch lengthways although it will stretch in width allowing it accurately to fit the limb.

A wooden spreader with a hole in the centre for the cord carrying the weight. The spreader separates the two lengths of strapping along the limb and prevents pressure on the prominences of the malleoli at the ankle. The strapping may enclose the spreader or may be fastened to it by webbing and buckles.

Extension cord and pulleys.

Padding for bony prominences such as the condyles of the tibia, head of the fibula and the malleoli. Folds of flannel, pieces of felt or wool may be used.

Crêpe, domette or woven edge cotton bandages, 3, $3\frac{1}{2}$ and 4 inches wide.

Safety-pins.

Tape measure.

Scissors.

Weights.

Requisites for shaving the limb should be provided, although some surgeons prefer to apply the strapping to the unshaved skin.

Method of Applying the Adhesive Strapping to the Skin

The width of the strapping used is from 3 to 5 inches, according to the size of the limb. It may be wider at the upper end and narrowed by being folded in at the distal end. The length of the two strips to be applied to the outer and inner aspects of the limb will be measured from the level on the limb indicated by the surgeon to about 3 inches below the sole of the foot. The last 8 inches are narrowed by cutting or turning in, and covered on the adhesive side with an 8-inch strip of plaster of the same width in order to provide a non-sticky surface in contact with the ankle. The edges of the long strips are snipped at intervals to allow the strapping to fit the limb without wrinkling. An alternative method is to cut the strapping lengthways in three narrow strips as far as the lower 8 or 10 inches, the three strips can be separated and, when applied to the skin, will lie more smoothly than one wide piece. The double thickness of strapping at the lower end is attached to the buckles of the stirrup or spreader. If the spreader is to be enclosed in the strapping then two pieces are cut, one double the length of the single strips referred to above, and a shorter strip about 10 inches long. The spreader is placed in the centre of the long strip against the adhesive surface. The second strip is placed, also adhesive surface down, over the middle section of the long strip so that both strips are enclosing the spreader and a non-sticky surface is provided wherever the strapping may come in contact with the ankle. A hole is made in the strapping to correspond with the hole in the centre of the spreader. A crêpe or woven cotton bandage is applied over the

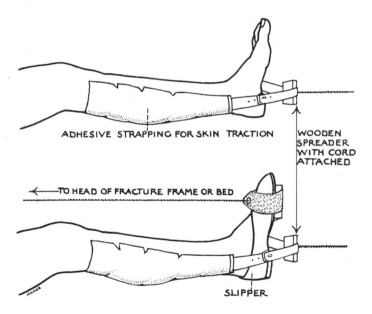

ADHESIVE STRAPPING FOR SKIN TRACTION

WOODEN SPREADER WITH CORD ATTACHED

←—TO HEAD OF FRACTURE FRAME OR BED

SLIPPER

Fig. 15.4. APPLICATION OF ADHESIVE STRAPPING FOR SKIN TRACTION AND METHOD OF APPLYING SLIPPER AND CORD FOR THE PREVENTION OF "FOOT-DROP".

strapping beginning at a point well above the prominence of the malleoli. A system of pulleys, cords and balancing weights is usually arranged to allow the patient to adjust his position. He is encouraged to exercise the muscles and joints by movement which can be carried out safely as the traction through the long axis of the fractured bone is constant.

Vertical Suspension with Skin Traction (Fig. 15.5)

This method is used in the treatment of fractures of the femur in young children under the age of six. Both the fractured and the sound limb are suspended vertically to a beam across the cot. The buttocks are lifted clear of the bed and the child's body acts as the counter-weight. In this position the child is easily attended to and the soiling of strappings or bandages is avoided.

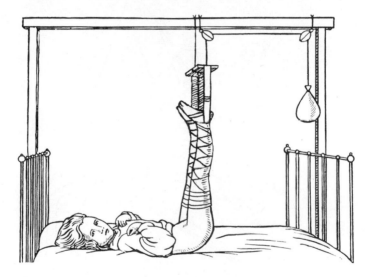

Fig. 15.5. BRYANT'S EXTENSION FOR FRACTURE OF THE FEMUR IN INFANTS AND YOUNG CHILDREN.

Note that the buttocks are raised from the bed, so that the body weight provides counter-extension.

Skeletal Traction

The insertion of the pin is carried out in the theatre. Steinmann's pin, which has a sharp point at one end and a nail head at the other, is hammered through the bone and the ends of the pin are held in a metal stirrup. Böhler's rotating stirrup is commonly used. The cord carrying the weight is attached by a hook to the ring of the stirrup. The sharpened end of the pin is covered with a metal cap or a cork. Denham's pin is similar to the Steinmann pin, but has a thread which grips the bone.

Kirschner's wire is inserted through the bone by means of a drill and the ends of the wire are held in a horseshoe metal stirrup. An S-shaped hook attached to the stirrup carries the weight cord.

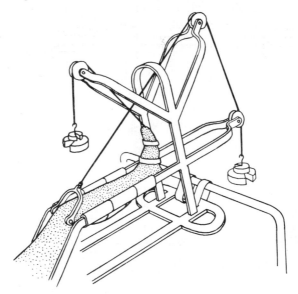

Fig. 15.6. SKELETAL TRACTION USED WITH A BRAUN'S SPLINT IN THE TREATMENT OF A FRACTURED FEMUR.

Kirschner's wire is not used as commonly as the Steinmann or Denham pin because the fine wire tends to cut through the bone. The skin around the pin or wire is dressed with sterile gauze, and sealed with collodion or Mastisol.

Weight. The amount of weight used for traction will depend on the fracture, on the weight and muscular development of the patient and on the type of traction used. An average weight for skin traction is from 4 to 7 lb. and for skeletal traction from 10 to

20 lb. Maximum weight may be applied for the first few days, in order to overcome the powerful contraction of the muscles, and later reduced.

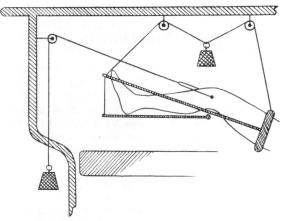

Fig. 15.7. LAYOUT OF TRACTION APPARATUS FOR TREATMENT OF FRACTURES OF THE SHAFT OF THE FEMUR.

The limb rests in a Thomas's splint. One weight holds the limb in balanced suspension from the overhead beam, while the other weight exerts continuous traction in the line of the femoral shaft.

(Adapted from *Outline of Fractures*, by courtesy of E. & S. Livingstone Ltd.)

Following the application of traction the nurse should attend to the following points:

(1) The weight must exert continuous pull. At no time should the weight be lifted or allowed to rest on the bed.

(2) The cord must run freely over the pulley.

(3) The foot must be supported and kept warm.

(4) Where a Thomas's splint is used the limb and the splint must swing clear of the bed when the patient moves.

(5) When skin traction has been used the limb should be frequently inspected to make sure that the adhesive strapping has not slipped or wrinkled (in which case it is likely to cause a sore) or that it has not broken.

(6) Pressure areas, such as the medial and lateral malleoli and the head of the fibula, should be well protected by padding.

16 OBSERVATION OF VOMIT, SPUTUM, URINE AND STOOLS: URINE TESTING: COLLECTION OF SPECIMENS

Observation of Vomit

Vomiting is a muscular action which results in the contents of the stomach being ejected through the mouth. The nerve centre from which the muscles concerned receive their messages is in the medulla of the brain, and this vomiting centre may be stimulated in various ways.

Peripheral Stimulation. Afferent messages reach the centre from outside the brain:

(1) as a result of irritation in the stomach, either due to some abnormal condition of the organ or to some irritating quality in the stomach contents;

(2) as a result of severe pain, especially of the "colic" type;

(3) as a result of an abnormal condition in the abdomen, *e.g.* intestinal obstruction;

(4) by a variety of stimuli, which will vary in individuals, as, for example, an unpleasant sight or smell, or the disturbance produced by the movement of a boat, aeroplane or train.

Central Stimulation. Nerve cells in the brain are directly stimulated by:

(1) Any condition in which the intracranial pressure is increased, *e.g.* cerebral tumour/cerebral abscess, meningitis, concussion.

(2) Poisons circulating in the blood, *e.g.* bacterial toxins, drugs, products of abnormal metabolism, or excess of waste products retained in the blood.

Note should be taken of the following points with regard to vomiting:

(1) Whether preceded by complaint of nausea or by retching.

(2) Whether the vomiting occurs at any particular time of the day, and if it is related to the taking of food.

(3) Whether it is associated with any particular article in the diet.

(4) Whether it is preceded by or accompanied by pain.

(5) Whether pain is relieved by vomiting.

(6) Whether the vomiting is forcible in character—"projectile vomiting".

(7) Whether the vomiting is regurgitant in character.

The material vomited should be saved for inspection and note made of the quantity of the vomit and the number of times vomiting occurs in twenty-four hours. Commonly the vomit consists of food or liquid recently ingested and mixed with mucus.

Bilious or green vomit is due to the presence of bile and is seen when the vomiting continues after the stomach has been emptied of food.

Dark-brown foul-smelling fluid is vomited in intestinal obstruction after preliminary vomiting of food and bile, it is often referred to as "fæcal vomiting".

Blood may be vomited as a result of damage to the stomach wall by ulcers, new growths or corrosive poisons, or from rupture of œsophageal veins. Blood may also be vomited if it has reached the stomach from the nose, mouth, nasopharynx or pharynx. The vomiting of blood is referred to as hæmatemesis.

Blood which has been in the stomach for a time is changed by the gastric juice and when vomited is a brown colour and is compared in appearance to coffee grounds.

Very profuse vomiting occurs in dilatation of the stomach, which may be a post-operative complication, and in hypertrophy of the stomach resulting from a narrowing of the opening into the duodenum (pyloric stenosis).

Hyperemesis is a term applied to persistent vomiting, and is usually used to describe the condition of exaggeration of the common morning sickness of pregnancy.

Observation of Sputum

Sputum is material which is expelled from the respiratory passages by coughing. Such material should be received into a sputum container, and, especially in infectious lung conditions such as tuberculosis, the use of handkerchiefs for the reception of sputum should be forbidden. The quantity and type of sputum should be noted, and also whether the patient expectorates it easily or if it is tenacious.

(For instructions in dealing with sputum and cleaning sputum mugs see p. 26, for collection of specimens of sputum see p. 212.)

Mucoid Sputum. This is clear mucus, tenacious in character, usually seen in the early stages of inflammatory conditions such as pneumonia or bronchitis.

Mucopurulent Sputum. A mixture of pus and mucus seen in the resolving stage of an acute inflammatory condition, and also in chronic infections such as tuberculosis and chronic bronchitis. In some cases it may originate in the nose or nasal sinuses.

Purulent Sputum consists of pus coughed up from dilated bronchioles (bronchiectasis), or from the rupture into a bronchus of a lung abscess or of an abscess in an adjacent structure.

Blood-stained Sputum. Rusty-coloured sputum is often seen in pneumonia, the blood has altered in colour and is mixed with the mucoid material. Streaks of bright red blood in the sputum may come from the gums or from congested mucous membrane anywhere in the respiratory tract. If the blood originates in the lung the sputum is likely to be coloured for several days.

Hæmoptysis is the term used to describe the coughing up of blood in any quantity. The blood is bright red and frothy. Hæmoptysis most commonly occurs in pulmonary tuberculosis, bronchiectasis and carcinoma of the bronchus. It may also be due to a pulmonary infarct, pulmonary congestion or to the rupture of an aortic aneurysm.

Fœtid Sputum. Extremely offensive material is expectorated in gangrene of the lung, advanced bronchiectasis and tuberculosis with cavity formation. Such sputum, if allowed to stand in a specimen glass, will separate into three layers. The upper layer is frothy, the middle layer turbid and the bottom layer shows a deposit of pus and shreds of tissue.

Abundant Frothy Sputum is characteristic of acute œdema of the lung, and may occur in cases of high blood pressure, cardiac or renal disease, asthma, or following inhalation of irritating fumes such as phosgene or chlorine gas.

Observation of Urine

Normal urine is a clear amber fluid with a characteristic odour, having a slightly acid reaction, and a specific gravity of 1,004 to 1,025. The specific gravity of urine is weight of 1 litre of urine compared with the weight of 1 litre of water which is 1,000 grammes. The weight of 1 litre of urine normally varies from 1,004 grammes when the urine is diluted as a result of a high fluid intake, to 1,025 grammes or higher when the urine is concentrated as the result of restricted fluid intake or excessive fluid loss by sweating.

The average amount passed daily is about 1,500 mils (52 oz.). Normal urine consists of water, urea and other nitrogenous waste, chlorides, urates, phosphates and a pigment of uncertain origin named urochrome.

The amount of water excreted varies according to the fluid intake and the needs of the body, the amount of salts excreted will also be a variable quantity but the amount of urea excreted in health on a normal diet is constant.

Collection of Specimens of Urine

Urine passed in the early morning is usually collected for routine testing as it is less affected by variable factors, such as fluid intake and food, than urine passed during the day. In all urgent cases and emergency admissions to the ward a specimen should be obtained as soon as possible, if necessary by catheterization. The urine should be measured and put into a clean specimen glass, covered and labelled with the patient's name, the date and time at which the urine was passed and the amount.

Collecting a specimen of urine from an infant is not always easy, but it can usually be obtained with a little ingenuity. In the case of a male infant a test tube or a piece of Paul's thin-walled rubber tubing can be placed over the penis and strapped to the anterior abdominal wall. A receiver or small bowl can be used for a female infant. As babies often pass urine while feeding, the receptacle should be put in position before starting to give a feed.

Urine for Bacteriological Examination. The specimen of urine must be collected with aseptic precautions into a sterile container. In the case of a female patient a catheter specimen may be required (see page 278). Catheterization, however, always carries some risk of infection and a "clean" specimen is often accepted in place of a catheter specimen. To obtain a clean specimen the vulva is carefully washed and then the area around the urethral orifice is gently, but thoroughly, cleaned, using sterile swabs and a mild lotion, such as 0·5 per cent. cetrimide. The patient is asked to pass one or two ounces of urine to flush the urethra. The flow is then interrupted, the sterile container is put in position and the mid-stream urine is collected.

Catheterization is seldom required in the case of a male patient. After preliminary cleansing a mid-stream specimen is collected into a sterile urine jar or urinal.

Specimens of urine required for bacteriological examination should be labelled and sent to the laboratory without delay.

Twenty-four Hour Specimens of Urine. Collection of all the urine passed over a 24-hour period may be needed in order to estimate the total volume, or may be required by the laboratory for investigations for *Mycobacterium tuberculosis* or chemical tests. Such specimens need not be sterile. All urine passed during the period, for example, from 8 a.m. until 8 a.m. the following day, is emptied into a large jar labelled with the patient's name, the ward, and the date. At 8 a.m. the patient is asked to pass urine, this is discarded; all urine passed during the next 24 hours is put in the collecting jar. At 8 a.m. the next morning the patient is asked to pass urine and this is added to that already in the jar. In some cases the entire contents of the jar are sent to the laboratory. Alternatively two specimens, containing some of the sediment from the bottom of the jar, and a record of the total measurement are required.

It is important that the 24-hour collection should be complete and for women patients two bed-pans may be needed to prevent contamination of the urine when the patient has her bowels opened. She should be asked to pass urine first and then be given the second bed-pan. If the patient is allowed to go to the W.C. she should be given a urine jar and instructed to pass urine into this.

Alteration in the Colour of Urine is usually due to concentration, but may be due to:

(1) Blood: when the urine may be coloured red or the blood may give it a smoky, dark appearance.

(2) Bile: when the urine varies from brown to a dark green or almost black colour.

(3) Certain drugs colour the urine, *e.g.* santonin, which gives an orange colour.

(4) Dyes excreted in the urine will alter the colour, *e.g.* a blue colour is shown after the injection of indigo-carmine.

Odour. (1) An ammoniacal smell. This is usually due to decomposition; on standing, the urea is converted by bacterial action into carbonate of ammonia. In cystitis the urine may be alkaline when freshly passed, and the odour of ammonia may be noticed.

(2) Acetone gives a sweetish odour which has been compared with that of new-mown hay.

(3) Infection with *Bacterium coli* gives a fishy smell.

Reaction. Normal urine is slightly acid.

The acidity or alkalinity of urine may be tested with red and blue litmus paper. Acid urine turns blue litmus red, alkaline urine turns red litmus blue. More accurate determination of the pH (the formula for expressing acidity or alkalinity of nearly neutral solutions) is made in the laboratory. Urine may be alkaline in cases of cystitis, if the specimen tested is stale, if the patient is on a vegetarian or very low protein diet, or if the patient is taking alkalis in any quantity by mouth.

Specific Gravity. This is recorded by means of an instrument called the urinometer. It should be allowed to float freely in the fluid in the specimen glass, and the figure is read off from the scale on the instrument, taking the lower level of the meniscus that forms round the stem.

A high specific gravity is found in concentrated urine and also in urine containing sugar.

A dilute urine gives a low specific gravity, a persistently low figure showing inability on the part of the kidneys to concentrate the urine.

Sediment. Normal urine may show a sediment on standing and cooling. This is due to the deposition of urates or phosphates, normal urinary constituents. Urates form a pink or red deposit in urine which is concentrated and acid. If the specimen or urine is gently warmed the sediment will disappear. Phosphates form a white sediment in alkaline or neutral urine. If the urine is acidified by the addition of a few drops of acetic acid the deposit will clear.

Abnormal substances which will form a sediment on standing are pus, mucus and renal tubule casts.

Notes on Urine Testing

Tests for Protein (Albumin)

"**Albustix**" **Reagent Strips.** The test end of the strip is dipped in the urine and removed immediately. If no protein is present the moistened end of the strip shows no colour change, but if protein is present a green or blue-green colour develops at once. Comparison with a colour scale provides a guide to the amount of protein present.

Hot Test. Fill two-thirds of a test tube with urine and boil the top inch over a flame, holding the tube near the bottom. A cloud appears on boiling which may be due to protein or to phosphates. Add a few drops of dilute acetic acid. If the cloud disappears, it is due to phosphates; if it persists or becomes denser, protein is present.

Salicyl-sulphonic Acid Test. To 2 inches of urine in a test tube add 10 drops of a 25 per cent. solution of salicyl-sulphonic acid. If protein is present, the urine in the test tube presents a turbid white appearance.

The Use of Esbach's Albuminometer for the Quantitative Estimation of Protein. The urine must be clear, not too concentrated and acid in reaction. Therefore, it may be necessary to filter or centrifuge the specimen, to dilute it and to acidify it before making the test. The test tube of the albuminometer is filled to the mark U with urine and to the mark R with the reagent (Esbach's reagent is a solution of 10 grammes picric acid and 20 grammes citric acid in 1,000 ml. water). Cork the tube, shake by inverting several times, and set aside for twenty-four hours. The height of the precipitate which forms at the bottom of the tube is read off on the graduated scale and indicates, approximately, grammes of dry protein per 1,000 parts. Divide the result by 10 to obtain the percentage of protein and allow for the dilution of the urine if necessary. Esbach's albuminometer should not be allowed to read more than 4 parts per 1,000; if, for example, it shows 10 parts per 1,000 the urine should be diluted. This test is not very accurate and quantitative estimation is usually carried out in the laboratory.

Tests for Blood

The presence of blood in the urine is usually visible to the naked eye. The presence of red blood cells is demonstrated by microscopic examination.

"Occultest". A sensitive test for the detection of blood in urine is provided by "Occultest" tablets. One drop of well mixed urine from the specimen is placed in the centre of the test paper and one tablet is placed in the centre of the moist area. Two drops of water are then added to the tablet. A positive result is shown by the development of a diffuse area of blue colour appearing on the test paper around the tablet within two minutes.

The Guaiacum test for blood pigment is occasionally used.

To 1 inch of urine in a test tube add a few drops of tincture of guaiacum and 1 inch of ozonic ether or ozonic alcohol. If blood is present, a blue ring appears at the junction of the two liquids.

N.B.—A positive reaction is also given by the urine of patients taking iodides.

Tests for Glucose

Benedict's Test. Benedict's solution is a solution of sodium carbonate, sodium citrate and copper sulphate. To 1 inch of Benedict's solution in a test tube add not more than 8 drops of urine and boil for two minutes. Allow to cool. A precipitate which may be greenish-yellow, yellow or orange will appear if glucose be present. Any precipitate appearing after fifteen minutes is of no significance.

"Clinitest" Tablets. "Clinitest" reagent in tablet form is particularly useful for diabetic patients who have to test their own urine at home as the procedure is simple and the results accurate provided that the tablets are fresh. Place 5 drops of urine in a small test tube using a pipette. Rinse the pipette, add 10 drops of water and then drop in one Clinitest tablet. Fifteen seconds after the boiling activity ceases in the test tube shake the tube gently and then compare the colour change with the colour chart provided. The presence of glucose is denoted by a green, greenish brown or orange colour according to the amount present. If an orange colour develops there is 2 per cent. or more of glucose in the specimen.

"Clinistix" Reagent Strips. These strips are impregnated with glucose oxidase and a colour indicator. The test end of a "Clinistix" is dipped in the specimen of urine and removed. If no glucose is present in the specimen of urine no colour change develops in the test strip. If the moistened end turns blue within one minute glucose is present.

Tests for Acetone

Rothera's Test. Take an inch of urine in a test tube and saturate it with ammonium sulphate by adding ½ inch of the crystals. Add a small crystal of sodium nitro-prusside or a few drops of a 1 per cent. solution, and then add ½ inch of strong ammonia. The presence of acetone is shown by a violet colour. This colour may not be fully developed for a few minutes.

Crystals of ammonium sulphate and sodium nitro-prusside may be supplied mixed in the right proportions in one bottle.

"Acetest" Tablets. The "Acetest" method is a convenient and accurate test for acetone and diacetic acid. Place 1 tablet on a clean surface, such as a white tile, add 1 drop of urine. Note the colour change at the end of 30 seconds and compare the colour of the tablet with the scale provided. A positive result is shown by a colour change which may vary from a pale lavender to a strong mauve colour.

Tests for Bile

Bilirubin

(1) Iodine test. Place some urine in a test tube and add a layer of 10 per cent. iodine solution. A green ring indicates the presence of bile.

(2) "Ictotest" Tablets. Place 5 drops of urine on the test mat provided and one "Ictotest" tablet in the middle of the moist

area. Add 2 drops of water to the tablet. A positive result is shown by the development of a bluish-purple area around the tablet.

(3) Fouchet's test. This is a sensitive test for bilirubin which is carried out in the laboratory.

Bile Salts. Hay's test. Put some urine in a test tube and sprinkle a little powdered sulphur on the top. The sulphur will sink if bile salts are present owing to the lowered surface tension.

Urobilinogen. Ehrlich's test. To 10 ml. of fresh urine in a test tube add 1 ml. of Ehrlich's solution. Invert the test tube several times to mix the fluids and leave for five minutes. The normal amount of urobilinogen will give a pink colour, abnormal quantities produce a cherry or darker red colour.

Tests for Pus

Microscopic examination for pus cells is the best test.

Observation of Stools

In adults the normal stool is solid or semi-solid, brown in colour and formed. The frequency with which a stool is passed varies in different individuals, but the average is once in twenty-four hours.

In infancy the normal stool is yellow and the bowels may act two or three times daily.

Fæces consist of:
Water.
Altered bile pigments, which give the normal colour to the stool.
Bacteria, mostly dead.
Mucus.
Cell debris from the intestinal tract.
Indigestible and undigested food.

Constipation is the condition in which the fæces are passed infrequently and are hard and dry.

Diarrhœa is the condition in which the stools are passed frequently and are fluid.

The bulk of the fæces will to a certain extent depend on the diet; on a mixed diet containing fruit and vegetables there will be a much greater bulk of residue than with a diet containing little residue such as a purely milk diet. Lack of fluids will also reduce the bulk in the large intestine.

In the ordinary healthy individual the bowels are usually opened after the first meal of the day, peristalsis being induced in the large intestine by the activity of the stomach and small intestine after a period of rest.

Note should be taken of the following points with regard to the stool:

(1) Number of times that the bowels are open in twenty-four hours.

(2) Colour, consistency and odour of the stool.

(3) Where an intestinal obstruction or paralytic distension of the intestine is suspected it is also important to note if flatus is passed, as the condition of absolute constipation in which neither fæces nor flatus is passed may be present.

The shape of the stool is probably of little importance, as this is altered by the anal sphincter.

False diarrhœa is the name given to the condition in which the patient has a fluid motion consisting mainly of mucus and very little fæcal matter. This may be noted in cases of carcinoma of the rectum and occasionally in old people in whom attention to the bowels has been neglected and a large mass of fæces is impacted in the rectum.

Putty-coloured Stools. If for any reason bile cannot enter the intestine, the stool will be light in colour owing to the lack of pigment. The stool will also be fatty owing to the lack of bile, and will have an offensive odour. The patient will probably be constipated.

The presence of undigested fat in the stool is found in jaundice owing to the absence of bile and in diseases of the pancreas where there is a lack of the fat-splitting ferment.

Tarry colour of the stool is due to blood which originates from high up the alimentary tract, either from the stomach or small intestine. The name given to this stool, which is composed almost entirely of digested blood, is "melæna". Very dark coloured stools are seen in patient's taking iron medicines.

Bright blood in the stool indicates bleeding in the lower part of the alimentary tract. The commoner causes are hæmorrhoids or piles, colitis, and carcinoma of the rectum.

Pus in the stool is due to the rupture of an abscess into the rectum or intestine, or to ulcerative colitis.

Mucus may be found in simple irritation of the alimentary tract following some indiscretion in diet or the use of a strong aperient. It may be present in large amounts in colitis and dysentery.

A collection of pus in the abdominal cavity, particularly in the pouch of Douglas, may cause irritation and congestion of the intestinal mucous membrane, and the fact that mucus is noticed in the stool may be the clue to the condition.

Foreign bodies of almost any kind may be swallowed, usually by children and passed in the stool. Such articles may take several days to pass, unless very small, being commonly held up to the pyloric orifice and at the ileo-cæcal junction.

The stools should be sieved until the foreign body has been recovered. The same procedure should be taken following an attack of gall-stone colic, as gall-stones which succeed in passing down the common bile duct into the intestine will be excreted in the stool.

Intestinal Worms. Roundworms, threadworms and tapeworms are the only intestinal parasites at all common in this country. If their presence is suspected, the stool should be collected in a bedpan containing warm water, carefully sieved through black muslin or any suitable thin material and any parasites or segments saved for inspection.

17 LABORATORY INVESTIGATIONS

Collection of Material for Laboratory Investigations

Examination and analysis of body fluids, excreta and tissues may be carried out in order to detect the presence of abnormal substances, an increase or decrease in normal constituents or, following the administration of diagnostic material, to assess the functioning of certain organs.

In a number of conditions bacteriological examination of urine, blood, sputum, serous fluid, and swabs from wounds or from the nose or throat is required in order to identify the infecting micro-organism.

In many cases the collection of specimens and the carrying out of the necessary preliminary preparation of the patient is part of the nurse's responsibility. She should fully understand her part in the investigation and carry out all instructions implicitly and accurately. Should any circumstance arise in which the carrying out of the full instructions becomes impossible, or if any error has been made this should be reported to the ward sister or the medical officer immediately.

The Collection of Specimens

All specimens sent to the laboratory should be as fresh as possible, for in many cases even a few hours' delay will render the specimen unsuitable for examination, due to bacterial decomposition or other causes.

All specimens must be clearly labelled to prevent loss or error.

Specimens should be collected first thing in the morning before breakfast, the taking of a meal may materially affect the level of some substances in the blood or urine. If it is impossible to collect blood samples before breakfast, an interval of at least 3 hours should be allowed to elapse between the last meal and the collection.

Specimens of Blood

When sending blood for examination the greatest care must be taken to avoid hæmolysis of the specimen, for hæmolysis almost invariably renders it unusable.

To avoid hæmolysis the syringe and needle used must be dry, so sterilizing in a hot air oven is recommended. The container into which the specimen is placed must also be dry and sterile.

For some tests blood serum is required, whilst for others whole unclotted blood must be sent. To prevent clotting potassium oxalate or sodium citrate is added to the specimen. Usually the laboratory supplies tubes with the required quantity of potassium oxalate crystals already added. If, however, these tubes are not available, 1 drop of 20 per cent. potassium oxalate solution should be added to the tube for every 5 ml. or part thereof of blood taken.

The chief exception to this is the blood sugar estimation, where a special tube must be used—this usually contains thymol and fluoride to prevent the disappearance of the sugar, which occurs very rapidly in unpreserved blood. Once the blood has been added to the anticoagulant it must be mixed gently—too vigorous shaking causes hæmolysis—but care must be taken to see that the anticoagulant is thoroughly mixed with the specimen. The specimen container must always be clean, dry and sterile.

Blood Specimens for Clinical Pathology

Bromide	..	..	..	10 ml. clotted blood
Calcium	..	..	..	*12 ml. clotted blood
Cholesterol	..	..	..	5 ml. oxalated blood
Chloride	..	..	..	7 ml. clotted blood
Carbon dioxide	..	..	..	*10 ml. heparinized blood
Cold agglutinins	..	..	..	7 ml. clotted blood
Cross matching	..	..	..	5 ml. clotted blood
Fibrinogen	..	..	..	5 ml. oxalated blood
Flocculation (liver) tests	..	..		7 ml. clotted blood
Gonococcal complement fixation test	..	..	..	7 ml. clotted blood
Kahn tests	..	..	..	7 ml. clotted blood
Paul-Bunnell tests	..	..	..	10 ml. clotted blood
Phosphorus	..	..	..	*7 ml. heparinized blood

* Special container and syringes for these specimens *must* be obtained from the laboratory.

Phosphatases	..	..	..	*5 ml. heparinized blood
Potassium ..	..	..	..	*5 ml. heparinized blood
Protein	..	..	..	7 ml. clotted blood
Sodium	..	..	..	*5 ml. heparinized blood
Sugar..	..	..	..	1 ml. fluoride blood
Thiocyanate ..	..	..	..	7 ml. clotted blood
Urea ..	..	..	..	5 ml. oxalated blood
Uric acid	..	..	..	5 ml. oxalated blood
Van den Bergh tests		..	..	7 ml. clotted blood
Wassermann reactions		..	..	7 ml. clotted blood
Widal tests ..	..	..	..	7 ml. clotted blood

* Special container and syringes for these specimens *must* be obtained from the laboratory.

Blood Counts

Blood counts may be made by drawing blood directly from a finger prick into special pipettes which the operator brings to the bedside. More commonly, however, venous blood is collected in an oxalate tube and sent, with two thin blood smears for the differential count to the laboratory for counting. This second method is more convenient, as several other examinations can be made from the same specimen if they are required. Usually 3 ml. are collected.

Normal Values

Red cells per cu. mm.
  Men   4·5–6 million
  Women   4·3–5·5 million
Hæmoglobin, in grammes per 100 ml.
  Men   15–16
  Women   13–15
White cells, per cu. mm.
  5,000–10,000
  Neutrophils   40–60 per cent.
  Lymphocytes   20–40   „   „
  Monocytes   4– 8   „   „
  Eosinophils   1– 3   „   „
  Basophils   0– 1   „   „
Platelets, per cu. mm.
  200,000–500,000

Erythrocyte Sedimentation Rate

The sedimentation rate measures the distance which the red cells fall in one hour when a column of blood is allowed to stand vertically in a glass tube of fine uniform bore. Several different methods are used, and the normal values vary with each method. It is not a diagnostic test as most infections cause an increase in the rate but it is very useful in following the course of a disease, *e.g.* in rheumatic fever and tuberculosis. The greater the activity of the disease the higher is the sedimentation rate.

Method. Wintrobe's method is the one most commonly used. 3 ml. of blood are placed in a tube containing ammonium and potassium oxalate, and well mixed. A special Wintrobe sedimentation rate tube is then filled and allowed to stand vertically undisturbed for 1 hour, and then the height of the column of clear plasma above the sediment of cells is measured.

Another method is the Westergren method, where 0·4 ml. of a 3 per cent. sodium citrate solution is used for the anticoagulant and a different size tube is used.

Normal Readings

	Men	Women
Wintrobe	0 to 9 mm.	0 to 20 mm. in one hour
Westergren	3 to 5 mm.	4 to 7 mm. in one hour

Bone Marrow Specimens

Samples of bone marrow may be required in cases of pernicious anæmia and leukæmia. These are obtained by puncturing the manubrium sterni or the iliac crest (see pp. 323–324), and aspirating the bone marrow.

Plasma Proteins

Disturbances of the serum proteins occur in many conditions. Abnormally low levels of serum albumin may give rise to œdema and may be the result of liver diseases, loss of albumin in the urine in the nephrotic syndrome or a diet deficient in proteins.

Serum protein levels are often low in patients with chronic infections or extensive burns.

Bacteriological Examinations

In many conditions specimens are required for bacteriological examination in order to identify the micro-organism responsible. Materials required for such examinations include:

throat and nose swabs
swabs from wounds
sputum
urine
fæces
blood
pleural and ascitic fluid
cerebrospinal fluid

These specimens must always be collected under strict aseptic conditions and in sterile containers. When taking swabs for bacteriological examination care must be taken to ensure that no antiseptic is applied to the surface for several hours prior to the swabbing. If the patient is under treatment by any chemotherapeutic agent at the time this should be stated.

Specimens will be examined by direct smear and by culture; information can also be obtained with regard to the sensitivity of organisms to the various antibiotics.

Swabs from the Throat and Nose, Wound Swabs

The necessary apparatus ready sterilized is usually obtained from the laboratory and consists of a swab fixed to a short stiff wire or stick, placed inside a test tube and sterilized. For nasopharyngeal examination special swabs in curved glass containers for passing behind the soft palate are supplied.

No antiseptic lotions should be used for swabbing or for gargles for four hours before the swab is taken.

Sputum

The best method is for the patient to expectorate directly into a sterile flask or small container with a screw lid.

If a sputum mug is used, it should be rinsed free from any trace of disinfectant and boiled.

Urine

A catheter specimen of urine or a "clean" specimen collected in a sterile container is usually required.

Fæces

A freshly passed stool uncontaminated by urine, is required. The specimen is placed in a container which should have a small scoop incorporated in the stopper.

Cerebrospinal Fluid

For complete routine examination 10 to 20 ml. of cerebrospinal fluid should be sent to the laboratory.

The following points should be borne in mind in collecting these specimens:

(1) Contamination with blood detracts from the value of the report in proportion to the amount present;

(2) Dilution of the fluid with water, saline, spirits and other fluids must be rigidly avoided;

(3) Bacterial contamination invalidates some of the tests such as sugar content and the colloidal gold test.

(4) The fluid is collected by lumbar puncture (see pp. 321–322).

Serous Fluids

Pleural effusions, pericardial effusions and ascitic fluid are formed in a number of conditions.

Microscopic, bacteriological and chemical investigations of these fluids are used to determine the nature of the underlying disorder.

(1) Cell content. In transudates only a small number of cells is present. In pyogenic infections pus cells are present in large numbers, while in tuberculous infection there is a high percentage of lymphocytes. Red blood cells are often present in malignant disease.

(2) Bacteriological investigations. In infective conditions culture for pyogenic organisms or the *Mycobacterium tuberculosis* may reveal the organism responsible for the infection. For the detection of tuberculous infection the fluid may be injected into guinea pigs.

(3) Chemical examinations. The protein content is increased in infective conditions, but may also be raised to a lesser extent in transudates.

Specimens of Tissues for Histological Examination

Specimens removed at operations should be sent to the laboratory as soon as possible.

Small fragments such as scrapings should not be allowed to become dried.

If the specimen cannot be despatched at once it should be placed for the time in a solution of 10 per cent. formalin in normal saline. Surgical or methylated spirit should not be used.

If sent through the post the nature of the contents should be stated on the label (*i.e.* material for clinical examination) and the parcel marked URGENT. There are special regulations relating to the despatch of specimens through the post, and special containers must be used.

Tests of Gastric Function

Tests of gastric function are used to estimate the hydrochloric acid in the gastric juice and also the amount of residual gastric contents after 12 hours' fasting.

(1) **Aspiration of Gastric Residuum** ("resting juice")

This test is carried out in the early morning after the patient has fasted for 12 hours. A Ryle's or Rehfuss's tube is passed (see page 232) and the entire contents of the stomach are aspirated, measured and saved. Gastric contents are aspirated at 10 or 15 minute intervals over a stated period, *e.g.* 1 hour. The fluid aspirated on each occasion is placed in a labelled test tube; each test tube is numbered consecutively. A hypodermic injection of histamine, 0·3 to 0·8 mg., may be ordered. Histamine stimulates secretion of hydrochloric acid, but in some types of anæmia there is no response to histamine.

(2) **"Tubeless" Test for Hydrochloric Acid**

This test depends on the hydrochloric acid in the gastric juice effecting an exchange of hydrogen ions with a dye, azure A, contained in the test substance. Azure A resin (Diagnex) is absorbed and excreted in the urine.

No preparations containing aluminium, iron or magnesium

may be given for at least 24 hours prior to the test; the patient
fasts for 12 hours before the test begins and nothing but water
may be given by mouth until the test is completed.

Procedure:

6 a.m.   The patient empties his bladder; this urine is discarded.
           He then swallows two capsules of a gastric stimulant,
           caffeine sodium benzoate, with a glass of water.

6.45 a.m. If ordered a hypodermic injection of histamine is given.

7 a.m.   The patient empties his bladder, the entire amount of
           urine is saved for the laboratory and labelled "control
           urine". The patient is given the Diagnex blue granules
           suspended in 60 ml. of water. The granules do not
           dissolve and the patient is instructed that they must
           be swallowed and not chewed. A further 60 ml. of
           water is given in the same glass to ensure that no
           granules are left.

9 a.m.   The patient empties his bladder and the entire amount
           of urine is sent to the laboratory labelled "test urine".

The directions issued by the laboratory should be carefully
followed and the timing must be accurate; if a repeat test has to
be done at least a week must elapse before the second test. The
patient will continue to pass blue or green urine for some days.

(3) Fractional Test Meal

The preparation of the patient is the same as for the gastric
residuum test. A series of specimen bottles or test tubes, one
marked "R.J" (resting juice) and the remainder numbered from
1 to 12, will be needed. An intragastric tube is passed and the
resting juice is aspirated, measured and saved. With the tube in
position, *either* the patient is given a meal consisting of gruel
made by boiling 2 ounces of fine oatmeal with one quart of water
until the volume is reduced to one pint; *or* alcohol (200 ml. of 5
per cent. or 100 ml. of 7 per cent. alcohol) is injected down the
tube.

At the end of 15 minutes the first sample of gastric contents is
aspirated (5 to 10 ml. is sufficient), thereafter a sample is aspirated
every 15 minutes until no material can be obtained. This procedure will take 2 to 3 hours. Each sample is placed in a numbered
test tube or specimen bottle and the whole series, with the resting
juice, is sent to the laboratory.

During the process the intragastric tube may become blocked; it can be cleared by pumping a little air down, using the aspirating syringe. The syringe should be rinsed after collecting each specimen. In the intervals the tube should be clipped and may be fastened to a towel round the patient's neck. If the patient is salivating freely he should be told not to swallow the saliva, but to spit it out into a receiver; he should be given paper handkerchiefs, or pieces of old linen, to wipe his mouth. This is a long and rather tedious process for the patient and he may be kept occupied by acting as time-keeper and given a bell to ring every 15 minutes.

Examinations of Fæces

Occult Blood

Meat, extracts and soups and very green vegetables, *e.g.* spinach, should be withheld for three days before collecting fæces for this examination; the administration of a purgative on the first of these days is recommended. Patient should not brush his teeth if this is liable to cause bleeding of the gums, but may use a moistened swab and a mouth wash. A sample of $\frac{1}{2}$ to 1 ounce of fæces is required.

The report states the result of the benzidene or guaiac test, a positive test indicates the presence of blood.

A quick test for the detection of blood in fæces is "Hematest". A thin smear of fæces is placed on the test paper provided, one "Hematest" tablet in the middle of the smear and two drops of water added. A positive result is shown by a diffuse area of blue colour developing around the tablet within two minutes.

Analysis of Fæces for Fat

It is of the greatest importance to inspect specimens of fæces before submitting them for quantitative analysis. The highly fluid stools obtained by means of purgatives and enemas are useless, as also are specimens which are non-homogeneous, unless these are thoroughly mixed to uniform consistency before sending the sample for analysis. It scarcely need be said that oily purgatives and liquid paraffin must not be used for several days before a specimen is sent for fat estimation. On occasions when the whole stool cannot conveniently be forwarded, the material available must be mixed to a uniform consistency and a 1-ounce sample sent in an airtight container.

The report states the percentage of water present, the percentage of the total solids which consists of fat (*i.e.* neutral fat, fatty acid and fatty acid as soap) and the percentage of the total unsplit fat.

Fat Balance Test

The patient is given a standard diet, containing 50 G. fat per day during the test and for at least 48 hours prior to its commencement. It is important that all the food should be eaten, but if any is left it should be returned to the diet kitchen. Liquid paraffin and oily drugs must not be given during the test, or for at least 3 days prior to its commencement.

Procedure:

7.00 a.m. 1st day. The patient is given 2 capsules of carmine (*i.e.* 1·0 G.) on an empty stomach.

7.00 a.m. 6th day. The patient is given 2 oz. of charcoal in water (*i.e.* 120 hours later).

Collection of fæces. The stools are examined as passed and those coloured by carmine are saved, as are subsequent stools until the charcoal appears; stools containing charcoal are discarded. The stools are collected in a sheet of cellophane placed in a bed-pan and covering the rim. The edges of the sheet are brought together and the whole stool in the cellophane wrapping is deposited in a large waterproof container.

In place of the full fat balance test, fat excretion on a normal diet may be measured over a period of several days. Normally, 91–99 per cent. of the ingested fat is absorbed.

Pancreatic Function

The internal secretion of the pancreas, insulin, is disturbed in diabetes mellitus, but is not usually affected by other diseases of the pancreas unless the organ has been extensively destroyed. This aspect of pancreatic function is considered under "Carbohydrate Metabolism" on pp. 221–222.

The external secretions of the pancreas may be tested either by estimating the amylase content of the blood or urine or by analyses of the duodenal contents for pancreatic enzymes and bicarbonates.

Urinary Amylase

A 1-ounce sample from a specimen of urine collected over several hours is desirable. When, however, it is a matter of urgency, as for example for the confirmation of a diagnosis of acute pancreatitis, examination of a smaller casual specimen is permissible. If the urine has to be sent some distance to the laboratory it should be preserved with benzene.

The normal range of urinary diastase is from 6 to 30 units per ml. A value of 200 or more units in a patient with acute abdominal signs is almost certainly due to acute pancreatitis. Intermediate values between 30 and 200, if found regularly may indicate pancreatic duct obstruction.

Duodenal Drainage

A more detailed examination of the pancreatic function may be carried out by examination of the duodenal juice obtained by duodenal drainage. A weighted tube (Rehfuss duodenal tube) is passed into the stomach and a specimen of gastric juice is withdrawn. The patient then lies on his right side to promote the passage of the tube into the duodenum. If necessary the position of the tube can be checked by X-ray. When the tube is in the duodenum the contents are aspirated and tested for sodium bicarbonate and the pancreatic enzymes, trypsin, amylase and lipase. Pancreatic secretion may be stimulated by a hypodermic injection of Mecholyl, or an intravenous injection of Secretin.

Liver Function

Tests of liver function are less satisfactory than function tests of some other organs because the liver has numerous functions, any single one of which may be deficient, whilst the others remain relatively intact. Also the liver has a large reserve and has to be very extensively damaged before any of the tests show an abnormal result. No test has yet been devised which tests the liver as a whole, but there are innumerable tests which depend on the different individual functions of the organ. The commonest of these tests are given below.

Bile Pigments

Failure of the liver to excrete bile pigments leads to the accumulation of these in the blood and their excretion in the urine.

Bilirubin. The normal level of bilirubin in the blood serum varies from 0·2 to 0·75 mg. per 100 ml. Increased serum bilirubin is found in liver damage, obstructive jaundice and hæmolytic jaundice.

Bilirubin will be present in the urine in all cases of jaundice except hæmolytic jaundice.

Urobilinogen. This pigment will be present in the urine in cases of incomplete obstructive jaundice, in diffuse liver damage, for example infective hepatitis and in hæmolytic jaundice. In cases of complete obstructive jaundice urobilinogen is absent from the urine.

(For urine tests for bile pigments see pp. 204–205.)

Serum Protein Tests

These tests are designed to show variations from the normal ability of the liver to synthesize serum proteins. They are not specific tests for liver damage since alterations in the serum proteins may be found in many other diseases.

In liver diseases the serum albumin level is low and the serum globulin is raised. The abnormal composition of the serum proteins is also reflected in the so-called "empirical liver function tests", for example the thymol turbidity and cephalin-cholesterol tests. These become positive when liver function is impaired, *e.g.* in cirrhosis of the liver and infective hepatitis.

Not less than 5 ml. of whole blood is required for each of these tests.

Bromsulphalein Test

This test measures the ability of the liver to excrete a dye, bromsulphalein.

The patient should have a fat-free breakfast and no food thereafter until the test is completed.

Procedure:

10.00 a.m. 5 mg. per kilogram of body weight of 5 per cent. bromsulphalein is injected intravenously very slowly over a period of 3 minutes. The ampoule must be warmed if any crystals are visible.

10.45 a.m. 10 ml. of clotted blood is collected from another vein, special care being taken to avoid hæmolysis.

Interpretation of the test. After 45 minutes the serum should show that less than 7 per cent. of the injected dose is still retained.

Prothrombin Concentration Test

Prothrombin is formed in the liver from vitamin K absorbed from the intestine. A low prothrombin may be due to liver damage, or to the non-absorption of vitamin K resulting from biliary obstruction. If the prothrombin concentration is low, the test may be repeated after an injection of vitamin K, and if it then returns to normal it is suggestive of biliary obstruction.

Liver Biopsy

This method of examination is described on pp. 324–325.

Renal Function

Chemical and microscopic examination of the urine, although valuable, gives only limited information as to the condition of the kidneys. Proteinuria, for example, may be met with apart from any nephritic condition, and in nephritis it is not always possible to form an opinion merely from a simple chemical urinary examination, whether the kidneys are functioning properly. Tests have therefore been devised with the object either of directly estimating renal efficiency or of investigating the severity and following the progress of events in a nephritic lesion.

Blood Urea Estimation
Procedure:

Breakfast may or may not be taken according to instructions.

8 ml. of blood is collected from a vein into a tube containing potassium oxalate to prevent coagulation.

If this test is done in conjunction with a urea concentration test the blood must be taken before the urea is given.

The normal range of variation of blood urea is from 20 to 40 mg. per 100 ml. Some authorities allow up to 60 mg. in elderly patients. Very high results of 100 mg. or more nearly always indicate serious renal impairment.

Urea Concentration Test (Maclean)

The intake of fluids should be restricted as much as possible from the afternoon preceding the test. No breakfast is given on the morning of the test.

The object of the test is to estimate the amount of urea excreted in the urine after giving a known quantity of urea by mouth.

A sample of blood for urea estimation is taken first. The patient is given 15 G. urea dissolved in 60 to 100 ml. of water.

The patient passes urine one hour, two hours, three hours and sometimes four hours, after taking the urea draught. The total amount of urine passed on each occasion is sent to the laboratory in bottles marked, " 1 ", " 2 ", " 3 " and if required, " 4 ".

Some authorities prefer to discard the urine passed during the first hour after the draught and consider only the results for the second, third and fourth hours.

A figure of 2 per cent. or over in one or more of the hour specimens is regarded as evidence of satisfactory renal function. Diuresis sometimes prevents this concentration being reached and if the volume exceeds 4 ounces (about 120 ml.) a concentration of urea below 2 per cent. does not necessarily indicate poor function. The restriction of fluids is designed to prevent diuresis and ignoring the first hour specimen (in which diuresis is often most marked) also aims at overcoming this difficulty.

Urea Clearance Test

The aim of this test is to estimate the efficiency of kidney function in relation to the average normal function.

Two methods are used, one without and one with urea, the idea of the latter being to impose a load on the kidneys to provoke maximum efficiency. The need for this is denied by some authorities.

At a stated time, *e.g.* 8 a.m. or 9 a.m., the patient empties the bladder. The whole amount of urine is placed in a bottle and marked " 1 ". A sample of blood is then taken for urea estimation.

If urea by mouth is ordered, this is now given.

One hour after the first urine has been passed the patient again empties his bladder and the whole amount is placed in a bottle marked " 2 ".

Tests for Carbohydrate Metabolism

Tests of carbohydrate metabolism are mainly used where diabetes is suspected or to check the diet and insulin dosage in patients with established diabetes.

Estimation of Blood Sugar

The specimen of blood is taken in the early morning before breakfast; 0·5 ml. of blood is collected into a tube containing a preservative mixture of sodium fluoride and thymol.

Where repeated estimations are required for a diabetic patient, all blood samples should be collected at the same time each day, the actual time being related to insulin administration and meals.

Normal fasting blood sugar levels are between 80 and 120 mg. of glucose per 100 ml. of blood.

Glucose Tolerance Test

If at all possible, the test should be carried out in the morning before food is taken. Smoking is forbidden. The patient empties his bladder; a specimen of this urine is saved and marked "A".

50 grammes of glucose in 100 ml. of water is given by mouth (the quantity will be less for a child, depending on age).

At ½-hourly intervals thereafter five more samples of blood are collected.

One hour and two hours after taking the glucose solution the patient empties his bladder. These specimens are placed in bottles marked "B" and "C".

The normal effect of a large· dose of sugar is to raise the blood sugar level in the first hour, but this returns to fasting level in two hours and no glucose appears in the urine. The diabetic patient may or may not have a raised blood sugar level before taking the glucose solution; after taking it his blood sugar will rise to above 180 mg. per 100 ml. and will remain above the fasting level for more than two hours. Although in the majority of cases glucose will not be present in the first specimen of urine, it will appear in the second and third specimens. Some people have a low renal threshold for glucose and in these cases glucose will appear in the urine after drinking the glucose solution, although the blood sugar remains within the normal range.

Calcium Metabolism

The commoner causes of disturbed calcium metabolism are diseases of the parathyroid glands and failure of absorption of calcium due to steatorrhœa or vitamin D deficiency and chronic renal disease.

In the condition of hyperparathyroidism due to tumours of the parathyroid glands calcium is lost from the bones leading to osteomalacia and a raised serum calcium level. In these cases the blood phosphorus is low and the alkaline phosphatase level in the blood is raised. In tetany due to absence of the parathyroid hormone blood calcium is low.

In steatorrhœa there is failure of absorption of calcium from the gut which gives rise to low blood calcium and osteomalacia.

The administration of vitamin D aids calcium absorption, but excessive dosage can cause a raised level of the blood calcium.

Laboratory tests used in disordered calcium metabolism include the following:

(1) Estimation of the blood calcium.

(2) Estimation of the blood phosphorus.

(3) Estimation of the blood alkaline phosphatase.

(4) Calcium balance estimation.

This latter test involves a somewhat complicated routine as detailed in the following instructions.

Calcium Balance Routine

The patient is on a weighed and analysed diet. The tray is delivered to the patient and collected by the dietitian, who weighs any rejects. The diet is the same throughout the test. The whole of it must be eaten. Nothing extra is allowed.

The water is distilled for drinking. As much as the patient likes may be given. All food is cooked in distilled water in utensils kept solely for this purpose. No toothpaste may be used, distilled water mouthwashes are substituted.

The patient is on this routine for 6 days before collections are begun. This is the equilibrium period during which time small alterations may be made in the diet to suit the patient's taste.

At 6 a.m. on the first day of the specimen collection, the patient empties the bladder. This urine is rejected. All subsequent specimens are collected in 24-hourly bottles, the last specimen of each 24 hours being obtained at 6 a.m. after which a new bottle is begun. Each bottle contains 10 ml. toluol to preserve the urine.

The evening before the start of the collections a carmine cachet is given to colour the fæces. This is given the evening before the end of each balance period. Following this all stools are saved in individual containers and the balance periods are considered to be from the end of the marked (red) stool to the end of the second marked stool.

Urine and fæces must be collected separately. The bed-pan is rinsed in distilled water before being used by patient. After use it is cleaned in the normal way and rinsed in distilled water again. All the fæces passed must be saved. The bed-pan is lined with cellophane to facilitate this.

No drugs may be given unless charted. All drugs given must be analysed. The advisability of giving any drug should be checked before administration.

This routine may be modified to allow balance tests on other substances to be carried out.

Phosphatase

Two forms of phosphatase enzyme are present in blood serum, the alkaline and the acid. The former is increased in bone diseases, such as hyperparathyroidism bone tumours and Paget's disease; the latter is frequently increased in carcinoma of the prostate gland with secondary deposits. The laboratory should be told which form is required when sending the specimen.

Either form of phosphatase can be determined on the serum obtained from 5 to 6 ml. of blood. The normal ranges vary with the method used for determination, and information will be given by the laboratory.

Tests of Thyroid Gland Function

Basal Metabolic Rate (B.M.R.)

At complete physical and mental rest a healthy individual consumes a definite volume of oxygen per minute, the actual amount depending mainly on the sex, age, height and weight.

During the test the patient lies quietly on a bed and breathes through wide rubber tubes into a special apparatus which records the respirations over a measured period of time, usually 6 minutes.

From the recording so made the volume of oxygen used by the patient can be measured. This is compared with the volume used by a normal subject of the same sex, age, height and weight.

Endocrine disorders, more especially those involving the thyroid and pituitary, profoundly alter this basal metabolic rate, and hence its determination is not infrequently of considerable value in detecting the existence and assessing the severity of these conditions.

The B.M.R. is considered normal if the figure obtained is within -10 to $+15$ per cent. of the value predicted for the individual in question. Success depends almost entirely on the patient being perfectly quiet and at ease; he must go without breakfast and should relax completely for about half an hour before the test is begun. This must be achieved without fuss about the test itself. In order to allay apprehension the simple nature of the procedure and its object should be explained, or, better still, demonstrated before hand.

Radioactive Iodine

A tracer dose of radioactive iodine (I_{131}) is given orally or occasionally intravenously, and the amount of "take up", or concentration of the radioactive material by the thyroid gland, is recorded by a Geiger counter sited over the thyroid area.

The results of the test may be invalidated if the patient is given radiological contrast media or food containing iodine, such as fish, thyroid preparations, perchlorates or thiocyanates, or radio-active isotopes. Some of these preparations may affect the result of the test even if a considerable time elapses between their discontinuation and the test, as for example Lugol's iodine and X-ray contrast media; it is therefore advisable to have an interval of 4 weeks if at all possible before carrying out the test.

The following instructions are usually given to the patient:

(1) No fish should be eaten for at least 2 days before coming for this test.

(2) Iodized throat tablets, cough linctus and any proprietary food said to have a high iodine content should also be avoided. If these have been taken during the past month, will you please inform the department at the time of making the appointment.

(3) A light breakfast may be taken on the morning of test.

18 THE USE OF INTRA-GASTRIC TUBES FOR FEEDING, GASTRIC ASPIRATION AND LAVAGE

Tube Feeding

General Considerations

Feeding through a tube passed into the stomach, either through the patient's mouth or nose is frequently required in the case of unconscious patients, in conditions where swallowing is difficult or impossible, for example paralysis of the soft palate or pharyngeal muscles, or after operation on the mouth or pharynx or larynx. This method of feeding may also be used in the case of premature or weakly infants who are unable to suck normally.

Any form of tube feeding is undertaken only on medical orders. In some cases the doctor may pass the tube; if it is the responsibility of the nurse she should have the help of a second nurse to check that the tube is safely in the stomach before the feed is given. If a fine tube is used there is a risk, particularly if the patient is unconscious, that it may be passed through the larynx into the trachea instead of into the œsophagus; should any fluid then be poured down the tube it will obviously enter the lungs, with disastrous, and possibly fatal, results. It is also essential to ensure that the end of the tube is not part way down the œsophagus but is actually in the stomach, as if it is in the œsophagus there is always the danger of fluid being regurgitated and inhaled. The usual method of checking the position of the tube is by attaching a syringe and withdrawing gastric contents. The aspirated fluid can be tested with a reagent, such as blue litmus paper which will turn red in contact with acid gastric juice. If there is any real difficulty in passing the tube, or doubt as to its position, the nurse should ask the doctor to verify that all is well before proceeding with the feed.

If tube feeding is continued for longer than 48 hours the diet must be adequate in calorie value and must contain the necessary food and accessory factors. Complan (see p. 104) is very commonly used and is suitable for patients of all ages and in most conditions; alternatively the feed may be milk with additions of soluble protein (casein) sugar, cream, butter or margarine, eggs, vitamin preparations, *e.g.* Marmite (vitamin B complex), halibut-liver oil (vitamins A and D) and ascorbic acid or orange juice to provide vitamin C. A fluid balance chart should be kept. Feeds are given at about body temperature, 38°C (100°F).

Frequent cleaning of the mouth should be carried out; this is particularly important in the case of unconscious patients. The patient who is conscious may be given pieces of orange to chew and spit out and mouth washes containing lemon juice and chewing gum; all these will stimulate the flow of saliva which is the natural way of keeping the mucous membranes of the mouth moist and healthy.

Feeding by the Nasal Route

The nasal route is more commonly used than the oral route; it is more comfortable for the patient as the tube can be left in position without causing him discomfort.

Requirements:

A small glass or polythene funnel.

A length of tubing about 8 inches to fit the funnel and a connector.

A suitable intra-gastric tube. For infants a size 4 catheter may be used, for adults a Jacques œsophageal tube size 6 to 8 (English gauge). A Ryle's duodenal tube is quite frequently used, but this tube is designed for aspirating stomach or duodenal juice and its fine openings are liable to block easily.

A large bowl for the apparatus.

Wool swabs or wooden applicators dressed with cotton wool to clean the nostrils.

A gallipot containing sodium bicarbonate solution for cleaning the nostrils.

A measure containing water.

A measure containing the feed.

A lotion thermometer.

A protective cape and a towel, or bib.

If a lubricant is to be used, either liquid paraffin or glycerin and borax are suitable.

A tray containing a tongue spatula, tongue forceps and a gag should be provided if the patient is unconscious, as it may be necessary to open his mouth in order to make sure that the tube has not entered the mouth from the nasopharynx instead of passing down the œsophagus.

A tray containing a 20 ml. syringe, an adaptor and litmus paper.

Method. The patient should if possible be sitting up. In the case of an infant or young child an assistant will be needed to restrain movements by wrapping the child in a blanket, and also to help by steadying the child's head. The cape and towel are arranged to protect the nightgown and one nostril is then gently cleaned, using a small swab wrung out in the sodium bicarbonate solution or the moistened applicators. The tube should be passed along the floor of the nose backwards and downwards. If the patient is able to co-operate, he should be asked to swallow, and then given time to take a breath before being asked to swallow again. A conscious patient will cough and splutter if the tube tries to enter the larynx; in this event the tube must be withdrawn and passed again. A deeply unconscious patient will not cough since the laryngeal reflex is lost, but he may become cyanosed if the tube is blocking the airway and this again is an indication for immediate withdrawal of the tube. When a sufficient length of tube has been passed for it to have reached the stomach, 16 to 18 inches in an adult, the 20 ml. syringe is attached and gastric juice is aspirated and tested as a check on the position of the tube. If all is then well, the œsophageal tube is attached to the tubing connected to the funnel and the feed is given fairly slowly, with the funnel held slightly above the level of the patient's head. When it is finished, water is poured down to clear the tube.

If the tube is to be removed it is disconnected, pinched tightly near the nostril and withdrawn in one quick movement. Usually, however, if tube feeding is to be continued, the tube is left in position and the free end is fixed to the patient's cheek, just over the malar bone, by a small piece of adhesive strapping. A spigot or a small clamp can be used to close the tube. Polythene tubes can be left in position for a week or longer if necessary; rubber tubes must be changed more frequently, *i.e.* after 24 to 48 hours. Polythene tubes also have the advantage of being easier to pass, since they do not bend or kink as the rubber ones tend to do. If continuous feeding is ordered, as in the "milk drip" used in the treatment of peptic ulcer, the tube is attached to a container with a drop counter (Fig. 18.1).

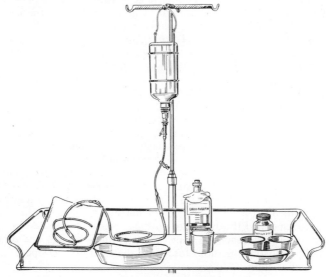

Fig. 18.1. EQUIPMENT NEEDED FOR CONTINUOUS INTRAGASTRIC "DRIP" FEEDING.

Feeding by the Oral Route

This is comparatively seldom used. The requirements are similar to those listed under tube feeding by the nasal route, except that a larger size œsophageal tube will be needed. The actual size used will depend upon the age, size and condition of the patient, and will vary from size 8 to 18, English gauge.

Method. In the case of an unconscious patient, he may be lying on his side or on his back with his head lower than his trunk. If he is wearing dentures these should be removed before the mouth gag is inserted. The tube is then passed over the back of the tongue into the œsophagus. A patient who is able to co-operate should be sitting up and as the tip of the œsophageal tube is guided over the tongue, avoiding the posterior pharangeal wall, he is asked to swallow, then given time to take a deep breath before he is asked to swallow again. Swallowing may be made easier if the tube is moistened and a large tube is usually more easily passed than a fine one. When 17 to 18 inches have been swallowed, the position of the tube is checked as described under feeding by the nasal route. If its end is safely in the stomach, it is then connected to the tubing attached to the funnel and the fluid is given. Afterwards a little water is poured down the tube, and when it is empty it is pinched tightly and withdrawn in one quick movement.

Feeding by Gastrostomy Tube

When the operation of gastrostomy is performed for the purpose of feeding a patient, a catheter (usually a self-retaining one, such as a De Pezzer catheter) is put into the stomach through an incision made in the abdominal wall and the stomach wall. The tube is taken out periodically and replaced by a new one.

It is especially important in the first few days after the operation to notice if the tube slips out of the opening, as it should be replaced at once. If it remains out for any length of time it may be very difficult to replace. Should the nurse have to replace it, she should remember the danger of pushing it between the abdominal wall and the stomach wall into the peritoneal cavity. The tube should be inserted without force into the centre of the opening.

Requirements:

Funnel.

Piece of tubing.

Tubing clip.

Connector.

A catheter, if the gastrostomy tube has been removed and the opening closed by gastrostomy plug.

Mackintosh.

Clean dressing and bandage, if likely to be required.

Measure containing water.

Bowl for apparatus.

If the gastrostomy tube has not been removed and the outer opening is closed by a spigot, a clean spigot should be provided to close the tube after the feed has been given.

The Feed. As the usual reason for gastrostomy is a malignant stricture of the œsophagus, the patient is probably emaciated from months of starvation. It is important that he should receive a diet which is adequate in nutritive quality and also containing the necessary accessory constituents of a balanced diet. A diet with a calorie value of 2,500 to 3,000 is desirable. The patient if properly fed, should regain some, at least, of his lost weight and strength, and keep some of his gain. Feeding is begun as soon as he recovers from the anæsthetic, and at first small quantities are given, but those are soon increased.

Any food that will pass down the tube may be given. Milk forms the basis, with the addition of eggs, cream, lactose and soluble protein, or complan may be used. Soup may be given with Marmite added for the vitamin B value. Orange juice given once a day keeps up the supply of vitamin C.

Method. The mackintosh is arranged to protect the dressing.

The spigot is removed from the catheter, or if the catheter has been removed the gastrostomy plug is taken out and the catheter required for feeding inserted into the opening.

The end of the connector is fixed to the catheter in the gastrostomy opening. The tubing is compressed to expel air. The feed is given slowly, finishing with water to wash through the catheter, if this is omitted the catheter may be blocked by coagulation of the milk as a result of the action of the gastric juice.

The connector tubing and funnel are removed and the spigot or the gastrostomy plug, whichever is used, is replaced. The gastric contents are very irritating to the skin should they leak through the tube, therefore a protective silicone cream, or similar application is applied around the gastrostomy opening. As soon as possible the patient is taught to give his own feeds.

Gastric Aspiration

Aspiration of the stomach contents, for diagnostic purposes or to empty the stomach, for instance in acute gastric dilatation or paralytic ileus, is usually carried out by a tube passed into the stomach via the nose, as described under feeding by the nasal route. A Ryle's tube or a fine œsophageal catheter may be used.

The gastric contents are aspirated by attaching a syringe to the

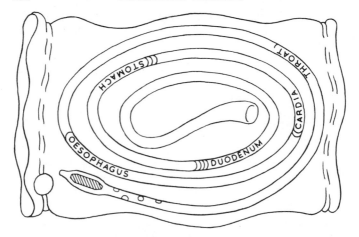

Fig. 18.2. PLASTIC RYLE'S TUBE.
Gamma ray sterilized in polythene bag.

end of the tube or by continuous suction using a siphonage
apparatus. A simple form of siphonage for this purpose is illustrated in Fig. 18.3. The intragastric tube is connected to a bottle
level with the patient's head. This bottle has a second connection
to a T-shape tube, one arm of which leads to a bottle suspended
about 3 feet above the bed level and the other to a bottle standing
on the floor. The suspended bottle is filled with water which
runs through the tubing to end under water in the bottle on the
floor; the flow is controlled by tubing clips. The rate of flow of
water from the upper bottle should be slow but sufficient to
create a partial vacuum in the bottle at bed level so that fluid from
the stomach is sucked into this bottle.

In cases where gastric aspiration is repeated, or where continuous suction is used, intravenous replacement therapy is
often required (see Chapter 20).

Gastric Lavage

Washing out the stomach is a procedure that may be ordered
in cases of pyloric stenosis, in intestinal obstruction immediately
before operation and in the treatment for poisoning when the

poison has been swallowed, particularly in cases of narcotic poisoning or acute alcoholic poisoning. A stomach wash-out may be given in the treatment of poisoning by a corrosive or caustic substance after the poison has been neutralized.

Requirements:

Jacques's œsophageal catheter, for an adult sizes 18 or 20, for a child sizes 8 to 14 (English gauge).

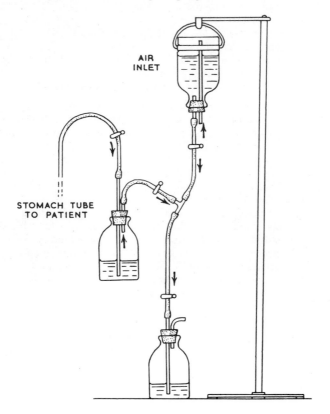

AIR INLET

STOMACH TUBE TO PATIENT

Fig. 18.3. CONTINUOUS GASTRIC ASPIRATION BY SIPHONAGE.

A connector.

A length of tubing (3 to 4 feet).

A large funnel.

Large jug containing the solution for the wash-out, *e.g.* tap water, sodium bicarbonate 1 drachm to water 1 pint, or normal saline 6 pints, which should be prepared at a temperature of 37·5°C (100°F).

A pint measure.

A large pail to receive the wash-out.

A receiver for tube after use.

A mouth wash and a few small squares of old linen.

A lubricant, such as glycerin, may be required.

A mackintosh to protect the bedclothes and a mackintosh cape to protect the patient's gown.

A gag will be required if the patient is unconscious.

Method. The apparatus should be placed in a bowl of hot water. The pail stands on the floor at the bedside and should be placed on newspaper to protect the floor. If the patient is conscious and able to co-operate, the usual position is sitting upright leaning slightly forward; if he is unconscious he may be placed in the prone position, with his head over the end of the bed or couch, or else on his back with his head lower than his trunk. The tube is passed as previously described.

The pint measure is filled with solution from the large jug and about 1 pint is allowed to flow in. When the funnel is almost empty, it should be inverted over the pail and the fluid syphoned back. The process is repeated until the fluid is returned clear or until the prescribed amount of the solution has been used.

The tube should then be tightly compressed and withdrawn quickly. A conscious patient should be given the mouth wash and the pieces of old linen to wipe his mouth. The contents of the pail should be measured and saved for inspection.

Several gallons of fluid may be needed to wash out the stomach in cases of poisoning. If unconscious the patient is placed in either the prone or Trendelenburg's position to prevent fluid running into the air passages.

19 OXYGEN THERAPY

Oxygen benefits the patient whose respiratory capacity is diminished, as is the case following chest injuries or operations on the lung, in pneumonia, acute pulmonary œdema, cardiac failure and many other conditions.

Oxygen Cylinders and Fittings

For purposes of identification oxygen and other medical gas cylinders are painted in distinctive colours and the name and/or symbol of the gas is stencilled on the cylinder. Oxygen cylinders are painted black with a white valve end.

Oxygen is compressed into cylinders of different sizes at 132 atmospheres, which is an equivalent of approximately 1,940 lb. per square inch. This pressure must be reduced prior to administration to a patient. Wherever possible an automatic oxygen regulator should be employed for this purpose, but when not available a fine adjustment valve may be used with care. A litre gauge or flowmeter is necessary in order that the prescribed rate of flow may be maintained. These gauges may be of the dial or the bobbin type. In the latter a bobbin inside a graduated glass tube rises as the oxygen passes through and the height of the bobbin against the scale shows the amount of oxygen being delivered. The flowmeter is usually incorporated in the cylinder fitting with the pressure gauge and regulator.

Before attaching the regulator to the cylinder the cylinder valve should be opened slightly, so that any grit or dust that may have accumulated may be blown out. The regulator is then fitted into the head of the cylinder by inserting the threaded end into the valve opening and tightening it by means of the winged nut. The litre gauge should be turned off and the cylinder opened slowly until the cylinder contents gauge shows "full", the cylinder is then opened completely by giving the key one more turn. The cylinder is then ready for use.

In some wards the oxygen supply may be delivered by a pipe-line to each bed, but every ward should possess at least one oxygen outfit ready for immediate use. The cylinder, in a wheeled stand with the fittings and the apparatus for delivering the oxygen to the patient, should be regarded as emergency apparatus which must always be kept in working order. An empty cylinder should be clearly marked "EMPTY" when removed from the stand and should be replaced at once by a full cylinder.

Fire Precautions

Although oxygen itself does not burn, any material which burns in atmospheric air will burn much more easily if the concentration of oxygen in the air is increased. Therefore certain precautions should be strictly observed.

Patients and visitors should be warned against smoking or lighting matches in the vicinity. No electrical bells, lights or heating pads should be allowed inside an oxygen tent and children should not be given mechanical toys. The patient must not be rubbed with oil or spirit whilst the tent is being operated; should such procedure be necessary the oxygen flow must be discontinued during the time that the treatment is being carried out.

Oil or grease of any description must not be used on the oxygen cylinder or fittings. The nozzle of the cylinder must be cleaned before attaching the regulator.

Administration of Oxygen

Oxygen may be given by means of a mask, an oxygen tent or through nasal tubes or fine catheters. Whenever a patient is having oxygen therapy he must be under continuous observation. The apparatus must be frequently and carefully checked; should the supply of oxygen run out, the patient may be unable to obtain sufficient air. In certain cases, for example in patients suffering from chronic bronchitis and emphysema who develop pneumonia, carbon dioxide may build up in the blood when the anoxia, which has been the respiratory stimulus in these patients, has been relieved. This can lead to carbon dioxide narcosis, the symptoms of which are a full bounding pulse, muscular twitchings, mental confusion and eventually coma. For this reason intermittent rather than continuous oxygen is usually ordered for bronchitic subjects.

Masks

The B.L.B. (Boothby, Lovelace and Bulbulian) Mask (Fig. 19.1). This apparatus consists of a rubber mask joined by a metal connecting device to a thin rubber bag similar to a football bladder. The usual type of mask is the oronasal one. The mask is fastened round the head by a rubber strap. Two tubes leading from the

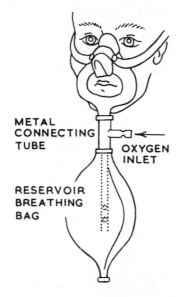

METAL
CONNECTING
TUBE
OXYGEN
INLET

RESERVOIR
BREATHING
BAG

Fig. 19.1. "B.L.B." Inhalation Apparatus (Nasal Type).

sides of the nose-piece pass round the sides of the mouth, joining over the chin to form a single tube to which the metal tube connecting with the breathing bag is attached. The connecting tube is fitted with an inlet tube for the oxygen. With a flow of oxygen at the rate of 7 litres per minute an alveolar concentration of 90 per cent. oxygen can be attained. The rubber bag has a capacity of about 700 ml., and should always be slightly distended while the apparatus is in use. When the patient breathes out, the expired air enters the bag and is mixed with the incoming oxygen. When the patient inspires, the mixture of air and oxygen in the bag passes through the connecting tube into the mask.

The face piece should be tried on the patient and the necessary adjustments made to the straps before the oxygen inlet is attached to the tubing connecting it to the cylinder of oxygen. Unless the situation is urgent, a little time should be spent in familiarizing the patient with the appearance and feel of the mask.

The nasal type of B.L.B. mask allows the patient to eat and drink and to expectorate while wearing it. If, however, the patient cannot breathe through his nose, or is unable to co-operate, the oronasal type of mask must be used.

Disposable Polythene Mask (*Oxygenaire*) (Fig. 19.2). This type of mask is light in weight and as it is inexpensive it can be destroyed after use and so presents no problems of sterilization. When the mask is connected to the oxygen supply, the flow of oxygen inflates a cuff round the edge of the mask, which then fits closely and comfortably. Should the oxygen supply accidentally run out the cuff will deflate, thus calling attention to the failure; in the meantime the patient can continue to breathe atmospheric air.

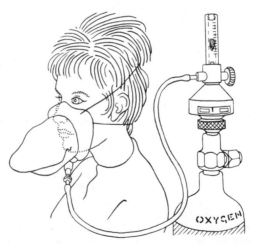

Fig. 19.2. DISPOSABLE FACE MASK (*Oxygenaire*).

The "Venturi" Mask (*Oxygenaire*) (Fig. 19.3). The Venturi mask is designed to give accurate control of the oxygen concentration so that it does not rise high enough to cause respiratory

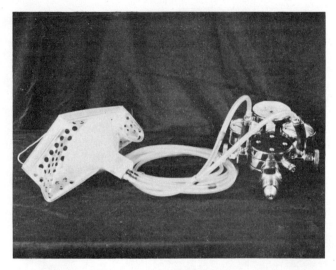

Fig. 19.3. A "Venturi" Mask (*Oxygenaire*).

depression, but is sufficient to relieve anoxia. The range of controlled concentration is 24 to 35 per cent. The disposable face piece is edged with foam rubber so that it fits closely and comfortable round the patient's nose.

Tracheostomy Mask (*Oxygenaire*) (Fig. 19.4). If a patient has had a tracheostomy performed it is obvious that he cannot benefit from oxygen given through a face mask. The tracheostomy mask shown in the illustration is made of perspex and fits over the tracheostomy opening; an opening with a peardrop cover in the front of the mask, over the tube, allows suction to be carried out with the mask in position. There are perforations at the side of the mask; these allow excess carbon dioxide to be removed and enable the patient to breathe atmospheric air, should the oxygen supply fail.

If a mask is not available, oxygen can be given by means of a catheter passed through the opening of the tracheostomy tube.

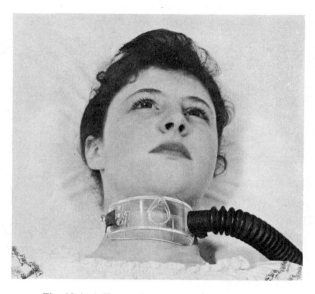

Fig. 19.4. A TRACHEOSTOMY MASK (*Oxygenaire*).

Oxygen Tent

There are several types of oxygen tents in use, but the general principles of construction and the management of the patient in the tent are very similar.

The aim is to have an oxygen content of 40 to 60 per cent. (average concentration 50 per cent.) inside the tent. The excess carbon dioxide must be removed, and the air prevented from becoming over-hot and excessively humid. The tent is made of transparent plastic material attached to a frame; the whole is mounted on wheels, enabling the tent to be easily moved. The windows in front are transparent in the other types of tent.

The canopy has openings, through which the nurse's arms can be put to give attention to the patient. Cooling of the air inside the tent is effected by passing the air through an ice box or through a refrigeration unit, and in some types of tents the carbon dioxide is removed by passing the air through a container of soda-lime.

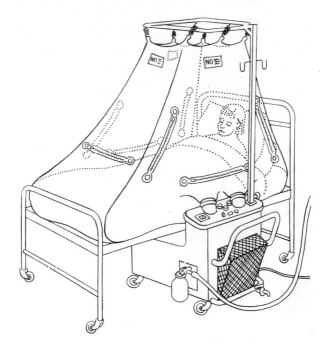

Fig. 19.5. AN OXYGEN TENT.

A full cylinder of oxygen ready for use, as described above, and a supply of ice should be obtained before erecting the tent. A wall thermometer will also be required. This is hung in the tent when it is erected, at the opposite end to the ice cabinet.

The ice is broken into pieces about the size of a man's fist and the ice container filled to capacity. About 3 feet of rubber tubing is then connected to the water outlet of the ice cabinet and a pail is placed under the rubber drain pipe. The ice cabinet is raised so that it will be clear of the ground when the canopy is fitted; the lid of the cabinet must be securely fastened otherwise there will be a leak of oxygen. A water seal is provided in the cabinet to prevent oxygen leaking through the drain pipe.

The head of the canopy must be securely attached to the openings provided on the ice cabinet, this is done by means of rubber inserts or rubber corrugated tubing. The back of the canopy has a nozzle marked "oxygen inlet" to which the rubber tubing from the cylinder regulator is attached. This should be done and the flow adjusted to five litres a minute before the canopy is placed over the patient. The temperature control should be set to "cold". Two persons are needed to fit the canopy over the patient's bed. The height of the tent and cabinet must be adjusted so that the head of the canopy will be from 6 to 12 inches above the patient's head. The skirt of the canopy is lifted and spread out so that it covers the bed and can be tucked in on both sides and at the back. The free end at the foot of the bed may be rolled into a sheet across the patient's knees. Alternatively, if a rubber sheet is placed over the frame of the bed the canopy is tucked in all round between the rubber sheet and the mattress. The openings of the canopy are closed with zip fasteners by rolling them up and securing the flaps with bulldog clips.

Once the tent is set up the oxygen flow should be turned on until the needle of the litre gauge registers "flush" and this full flow is then allowed to continue for about 5 minutes, after which time the flow is reduced to the dosage ordered, which may be from 4 to 8 litres per minute.

When the canopy has been opened to allow access to the patient the tent should be flushed with oxygen as soon as the openings are closed again. The temperature in the tent should usually be maintained at 18° to 21°C (65° to 70°F).

In some cases the patient may not be nursed continually in the tent; as already mentioned, certain patients suffering from respiratory disease may develop carbon dioxide narcosis if they are continually breathing a high concentration of oxygen. An example of the routine that may be followed in such cases is 10 minutes in the tent and 20 minutes with the tent open.

Caution is needed in the use of an oxygen tent for premature infants since high concentrations can lead to a condition known as retrolental fibroplasia and blindness. The minimum concentration of oxygen that will relieve cyanosis and respiratory difficulty should be given.

When an oxygen tent is dismantled after use the canopy should be mopped with a disinfectant, such as Savlon 1 in 20 solution, and then washed with soap and water.

Nasal Tubes

This method is used if a tent is not available or a face mask is not suitable, as, for example, where there are facial injuries. It is much less efficient than either the tent or the mask as it is wasteful of oxygen and the patient cannot as a rule tolerate a rate of flow greater than 4 litres per minute. Three types of apparatus can be used:

1. A bifurcated metal tube with two pieces of soft rubber tubing attached. The metal tube is carried by a head piece and webbing band which is fastened round the patient's head.

2. A spectacle frame which carries two pieces of rubber tubing and is worn by the patient in the same way as an ordinary pair of spectacles.

3. Two soft rubber catheters connected by a Y-shaped connection to the delivery tube from the oxygen apparatus.

When giving oxygen by nasal tubes it is necessary to moisten the oxygen by passing it through a humidifier before it reaches the patient, as dry oxygen is irritating to the nasal passages.

Before the tubes are inserted the nostrils should be cleaned with warm sodium bicarbonate lotion and wool swabs. A cocaine spray or cocaine ointment may be used in order to make the treatment less uncomfortable for the patient. The two nasal tubes should be passed about 2 inches along the floor of the nostrils. The tubes should be removed and cleaned if left in for more than twenty-four hours.

20 FLUID AND ELECTROLYTE BALANCE

The rapidity with which death can follow complete deprivation of water must have been part of man's experience since the beginning of human life and in medicine the necessity of replacing lost body fluid has long been appreciated in the treatment of such conditions as hæmorrhage, extensive burns, severe vomiting and diarrhœa. Only comparatively recently, however, has the essential role played in normal body chemistry by the various substances in solution in the water in the various compartments of the body been fully realized. The term "dehydration" as now used usually denotes loss of electrolytes, *i.e.* sodium, potassium and chloride, as well as fluid loss.

In health the amount of fluid in the body and its composition remains remarkably constant in spite of variations in intake, but in almost every case of serious illness or extensive surgical operation the balance can be gravely disturbed and its restoration may become a matter of urgency. For this reason one of the nurse's most valuable contributions to the treatment of the patient is an accurate 24-hour record of all fluid going into the patient and all fluid output, including the volume, the route and the type of fluid.

The Water Content of the Body

The total quantity of water in the adult body amounts to approximately 70 per cent. of the total body weight. Two-thirds of this water is inside the cells, intracellular fluid, one-third is outside the cells, the extracellular fluid; most of the latter is contained in the blood plasma and the interstitial fluid, lymph, which bathes the tissue cells. An adult weighing 70 kilograms (11 stone) contains in his body about 49 litres of fluid weighing 49 kg.; of this total about 31·5 litres are intracellular fluid and 17·5 litres are extracellular. Approximately 5 per cent. of the total body weight is accounted for by the water content of the blood, *i.e.* 3·5 litres.

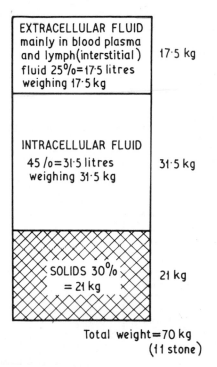

Fig. 20.1. PROPORTIONS OF FLUID AND SOLIDS IN THE ADULT BODY.

Substances in Solution: Electrolytes

Many substances are contained in solution in the body fluids; some of these, such as glucose, provide food for the cells; others, such as urea, are the waste products of cell metabolism and must be removed in solution in the water surrounding each cell. The interstitial fluid must be able to effect an exchange with the blood plasma as well as with the intracellular fluid in order to transfer to the cell those substances that it needs and to clear waste products from the cell into the blood.

Both intracellular and extracellular fluid also contain salts in

solution whose presence in the correct concentration is responsible
for the interchange of material through the semi-permeable
membrane which forms the cell boundary and maintains the
normal tension within the cell. These all-important salts form
what are known as electrolytes because in solution they dis-
sociate into electrically charged particles, or ions. Some ions
carry a positive charge and are known as cations, others are

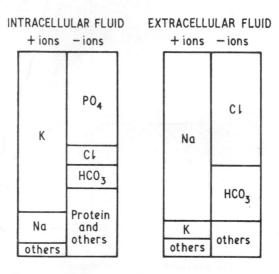

Fig. 20.2. COMPARISON OF ELECTROLYTES IN THE INTRACELLULAR
AND THE EXTRACELLULAR FLUID.

negatively charged and are called anions. The chief cations in the
body fluids are sodium (Na), potassium (K), calcium (Ca), and
magnesium (Mg). The chief anions are chloride (Cl), bicarbonate
(HCO_3) and phosphate (PO_4). The electrolytes in the extracellular
fluid are mainly sodium and chloride, while the intracellular fluid
contains mainly potassium and phosphate and little chloride.

The concentration of electrolytes in the body fluids can be
measured and is usually expressed by the biochemist in units
known as milliequivalents per litre (mEq/l). One mEq is a

thousandth part of the equivalent weight of a substance, equivalent weight being the weight in grammes equivalent to 1·008 g. hydrogen in a chemical reaction, or to the equivalent weight of any other substance. This figure therefore expresses not the actual weight of the substance in solution but its chemical combining power. To give one example of the chemical use of these calculations, the normal value for potassium in the blood plasma is 4·5 mEq/l. In some conditions, including acute renal failure, it is essential to check the blood potassium level; if it rises to 7 mEq/l or higher there is grave danger of cardiac arrest.

Acid-Base Balance

The maintenance of the normal reaction of both the extracellular and the intracellular fluid in terms of acidity or alkalinity is another factor which governs the health of the cells. The reaction of the extracellular fluid is normally slightly alkaline and this is expressed as a pH value of about 7·4, a range of 7·35 to 7·45 on this scale being within normal limits. Intracellular fluid is slightly acid but its reaction is not known precisely. The pH formula gives the concentration of hydrogen ions in solution; acid solutions have a higher concentration of these ions than alkaline solutions. The pH scale runs from 0 to 14, the higher the hydrogen ion concentration the lower the reading; 7 represents neutrality; if a solution gives a reading below this figure it is acid, above 7 the solution is alkaline.

The reaction of both extracellular and intracellular fluids remains virtually constant in health. Urine however has a variable reaction and although usually slightly acid, it can vary between 4·7 and 8. This is because one of the main functions of the kidneys is to maintain the normal reaction of the body fluids and to excrete any excess of either acid or base. The terms "acidosis" and "alkalosis" are frequently used and denote in the first case that the blood contains more acid than normal, and in the second that it contains an excess of base.

Daily Requirements for Water and Electrolytes

An adult excretes about 1 litre of urine in 24 hours and also loses about 1 litre through the lungs in expired air, through the skin as perspiration, and in the water content of fæces. He therefore needs to take in at least 2 litres of fluid daily to make good this loss. No harm results from an excessive intake in health as the kidneys are well able to dispose of unwanted fluid, a fact with which everyone is familiar. If there is an excessive loss of water, for example from heavy sweating, this will normally be made good almost immediately as the individual feels thirsty and drinks freely.

The minimal requirement of sodium chloride is not known, but the average intake of 59 (80 mEq) represents an enormous excess over the minimum. We are therefore not likely to be deficient of this in health since we all take common salt with our food. Potassium and other salts are also present in sufficient amounts in a normal dietary. In illness both water and salt often need to be given intravenously. For short periods no potassium is needed, but if no food is taken for more than a few days some potassium may be given, usually by mouth in the form of Mixture of Potassium Citrate, N.F., 30 ml., as when given by this route there is less risk of overloading with potassium.

In many conditions diminished intake is accompanied by excessive loss of water and electrolytes, for example by vomiting, diarrhœa, gastric aspiration, polyuria, plasma or blood loss. Treatment must therefore be planned to cover this loss as well as the lowered intake and allowances must be made for losses which have occurred before treatment started. Accurate intake and output records and repeated blood electrolyte estimations are essential features of successful replacement therapy.

Treatment of Fluid and Electrolyte Disturbance

In practice these disturbances are usually multiple, affecting the water content, electrolytes and acid-base balance simultaneously. For clarity of description, however, it is convenient to consider separately the most important factors and their appropriate treatment.

1. Water

(a) *Water depletion*. This may be due to excessive loss, diminished intake, or a combination of both; loss of fluid may not be obvious, for example in intestinal obstruction when large quantities can collect in the distended intestine and go undetected. Depletion due to lowered intake is particularly liable to occur in comatose or semi-comatose patients. Lack of water is characterized by thirst, dry mouth and tongue and decreased urinary output. In severe cases, where it is usually accompanied by sodium deficiency, the patient has a pale, anxious face with sunken eyes, the extremities are cold and may be cyanosed, the skin loses its elasticity, and in infants the fontanelle is depressed. The pulse rate is then usually increased and the blood pressure low. Water depletion can be corrected by giving fluid by mouth or by intra-gastric tube if the patient's condition permits, or by the intra-venous administration of a 5 per cent. glucose solution in water. In cases with accompanying electrolyte loss, however, the type of fluid to be given will be determined after estimation of the blood electrolytes.

(b) *Excess of water*. Excess of water, or "water intoxication", usually results from the administration of large quantities of fluids to patients whose urinary output is inadequate. The effects of water intoxication are due to increased tension within the cells and the clinical manifestations are mental confusion, convulsions and coma. The condition can be produced by the rectal adminis-tration of tap water or glucose solutions. Water intoxication can be prevented if an accurate intake and output chart is kept and if the fluid given is restricted, in the case of an adult, to a maximum of 1 litre plus the volume of the urinary output over the previous 24 hours. If the symptoms are severe the condition may be treated by rigorous water restriction, and occasionally by the intravenous administration of hypertonic (5 per cent.) sodium chloride solution.

2. Sodium

(a) *Sodium depletion*. Depletion may occur as a result of pro-longed vomiting, gastric or intestinal aspiration or drainage, diarrhœa, excessive loss of salt in the urine as in the polyuria of diabetic ketosis in Addison's disease and in some cases of chronic nephritis. It is characterized by loss of elasticity of the skin, low intraocular pressure and, when severe, by low blood pressure, circulatory failure and shock. Sodium loss can be made good by the administration of salt by mouth or intravenous infusion of isotonic saline solution.

(b) *Sodium excess*. Excess may be present in cardiac failure and in the nephrotic syndrome; it may be produced by the adminis-tration of large doses of cortisone or intravenous infusion of saline given rapidly or in excessive amounts. The effect of sodium excess is to cause œdema, which is most dangerous when it affects the lungs.

3. Potassium

(a) *Potassium deficiency* (*hypokalæmia*). Lack of potassium may be due to a low intake, persistent vomiting, diarrhœa, chronic renal disease, diabetic ketosis, excessive administration of cortisone, or occasionally to an adrenal tumour secreting aldosterone. The chief manifestations of potassium lack are muscular weakness, intestinal paralysis and myocardial failure. The deficiency may be made good by the administration of potassium by mouth in the form of potassium chloride or potassium citrate. 15 ml. of Mixture of Potassium Citrate, N.F., contains 3 g. of potassium (28 mEq). Potassium can also be given intravenously as 0·2 or 0·3 per cent. solution of potassium chloride, provided that the urinary output is adequate and that the rate of administration does not exceed 1 litre in 24 hours.

(b) *Potassium excess* (*hyperkalæmia*). Potassium excess occurs in cases of anuria from any cause and in Addison's disease of the adrenal cortex. Where hyperkalæmia exists there is grave danger of cardiac arrest, therefore in the above-mentioned conditions it is necessary to avoid giving potassium in any form.

4. Bicarbonate

Changes in the bicarbonate (HCO_3) content of the plasma reflect disturbances in the acid-base balance of the body fluids.

(a) *Acidosis*. In this condition there is a tendency for the pH of the blood to fall. This may be due to the formation of acids (ketones) as in diabetic ketosis, the administration of acid-forming substances, such as salicylates, or decreased excretion of acid metabolites in renal failure. Acidosis may also result from excessive loss of sodium and potassium, for example in cases of diarrhœa. In chronic respiratory disease, such as chronic bronchitis and emphysema, acidosis can occur from retention of carbon dioxide. Non-respiratory acidosis causes hyperventilation with deep sighing respirations, the "acidotic breathing" seen in diabetic coma and uræmia, and leads to mental confusion and coma. Treatment consists of the appropriate therapy for the underlying condition, *e.g.* the administration of insulin in diabetic

SOLUTIONS USED IN INTRAVENOUS REPLACEMENT THERAPY

Solution	gramme/litre	Na	K	Cl	HCO₃ equivalent
			(m.Eq./litre)		
5 per cent. glucose	Glucose 50				
Normal saline	Na Cl 9	155		155	
½ normal saline	Na Cl 4·5	77		77	
Glucose in ⅕th normal saline	{ Glucose 43, Na Cl 1·8	31		31	
Hypertonic saline:					
a. 2 per cent.	Na Cl 20	343		343	
b. 3 per cent.	Na Cl 30	515		515	
c. 5 per cent.	Na Cl 50	855		855	
⅛th molar sodium lactate	Na lactate 18·7	167			167
Saline lactate	{ Na Cl 5·85, Na lactate 3·39	130		100	30
Potassium chloride in 2·5 per cent. glucose:					
a. 0·2 per cent.	K Cl 2, glucose 25		27	27	
b. 0·3 per cent.	K Cl 3, glucose 25		40	40	
Sodium and potassium chloride with lactate	{ Na Cl 3·48, K Cl 3, Na lactate 4·48	100	40	100	40
Glucose electrolyte (for diabetic ketosis)	{ Na Cl 1·17, K Cl 1·49, Mg Cl 0·24, K₂ HPO₄ 0·87, Glucose 50	20	30	45	

HCO_3 equivalent; $K_2 HPO_4$

coma, and in chronic renal failure by giving sodium bicarbonate or sodium citrate by mouth or isotonic saline solution intravenously. Alternative solutions for intravenous therapy are molar lactate or saline lactate solution, with or without potassium according to the needs of the individual case.

(b) *Alkalosis*. In this condition there is a tendency for the blood to become more alkaline than normal. Alkalosis may be due to excessive and prolonged administration of alkalis or to loss of hydrochloric acid from persistent vomiting or gastric aspiration. The amount of bicarbonate in the blood plasma increases and the clinical signs are anorexia, mental confusion and sometimes tetany; long-standing alkalosis may produce renal failure. The treatment of this condition is intravenous isotonic saline solution; if renal function is normal the kidneys will retain the chloride and excrete the sodium. Potassium deficiency usually complicates alkalosis and this needs to be corrected simultaneously.

21 SUBCUTANEOUS AND INTRAVENOUS INFUSIONS; BLOOD AND PLASMA TRANSFUSIONS

In the preceding chapter some of the conditions in which replacement of fluid and electrolytes forms an essential part of medical treatment have been discussed. In some cases the loss can be made good by oral administration of fluids or, if the patient is unable to swallow, for example the unconscious patient, feeding by intragastric tube may be entirely satisfactory. Rectal infusion is another method of giving fluid that may be used, but this is not very reliable as the amount absorbed is uncertain and there is a risk of producing water intoxication since the patient cannot say when he has had enough; however, rectal administration may be a useful supplementary route on occasions, provided that the rate of infusion is slow (see pages 271–272). Parenteral administration is regarded as the most precise and controlled method of replacing or correcting fluid or electrolyte imbalance. The term "parenteral" means other than through the alimentary tract and includes infusion into the subcutaneous tissues, or transfusions directly into the blood stream; in the latter case usually into the venous circulation, but occasionally intra-arterially.

SUBCUTANEOUS INFUSION

Subcutaneous infusion of solutions is a method that is more commonly used for infants and young children than for adults. The solution used contains not less than 0·5 per cent. sodium chloride, 2·5 per cent. glucose solution may be added; stronger glucose solutions are liable to cause tissue damage.

Possible sites for subcutaneous infusion are the outer aspects of the thighs, the axillæ and the areas below the breasts; the infusion is given into two areas simultaneously. The rate of absorption

from subcutaneous tissue is slow but can be assisted by the injection of hyaluronidase (Hyalase). Nevertheless often not more
than 120 ml. (4 fl. oz.) can be given into each site without producing marked local distension and blanching of the skin.
Subcutaneous infusion is therefore mainly a method of supplementing the fluid intake and cannot be substituted for intravenous therapy in cases where replacement of lost fluid is urgent,
as in shock, when the superficial circulation is much reduced.

Subcutaneous infusions may be given with a 20 or 30 ml.
syringe and a fine needle about $2\frac{1}{2}$ inches long. The injection can
be made wherever a large fold of loose skin can be picked up; the
needle is inserted into the base of the fold and as the piston of the
syringe is gradually pushed home the needle is pushed further
into the tissues. More commonly, however, the fluid is given by
the gravity method as a continuous drip. For this procedure the
following will be needed:

    (1) Container with the sterile solution for infusion, connecting
        tubing, drip chamber, Y-shaped connection and tubing to
        fit the two arms of the "Y", adaptors and two fine sub-
        cutaneous needles, $2\frac{1}{2}$ or 3 inches long, three tubing clips.
    (2) Ampoules of Hyalase, 1 ml. syringe and needle for injec-
        tion.
    (3) Small sterile pack containing towel, swabs and gauze.
    (4) Dressing forceps.
    (5) Cetrimide or other skin cleansing agent.
    (6) Adhesive strapping and scissors.
    (7) Receptacles for used instruments and other articles.

The bung of the container is pierced by an air inlet tube and a
delivery tube, the container is then suspended on the transfusion
stand and the tubing clips are opened to allow the fluid to run
through the apparatus and expel air. The clips are then closed, the
skin of the areas chosen for the infusion is cleaned and a fold of
tissue is picked up in the left hand while the needle is inserted
with the right hand into the base of the fold and pushed in an
upward direction for its entire length. This procedure is repeated
with the second needle and the infusion is then started. When it
is satisfactorily established, 0·5 ml. Hyalase is injected into each
of the two pieces of tubing attached to the needles. The rate of
flow will need to be adjusted according to the rate of absorption
and will usually be the maximum rate that can be tolerated with-

out the formation of hard swellings and blanching of the skin at the sites of the infusion. The needles should be firmly secured in position by adhesive strapping. Clothing is not replaced over the

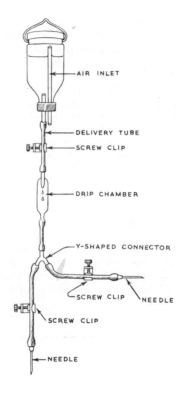

Fig. 21.1. SUBCUTANEOUS INFUSION APPARATUS.

sites of the infusion but the area is covered with a piece of cotton wool or Gamgee tissue, which permits easy inspection and at the same time keeps the patient warm.

INTRAVENOUS THERAPY

Intravenous Infusion of Electrolyte Solutions

Replacement of large amounts of fluid lost from the body or the correction of serious electrolyte imbalance is most rapidly and accurately dealt with by the introduction of a suitable solution directly into the venous circulation. Sodium chloride and glucose are the two most commonly used solutions. Examples of other intravenous solution used are Darrow's sodium potassium chloride lactate solution and dilute plasma with potassium chloride used in the treatment of fluid and electrolyte loss in infants. Electrolyte solutions are also given intravenously in the treatment of a number of conditions, for example diabetic coma and obstruction of the gut; in these cases the solutions are individually prescribed and carefully checked during treatment by frequent blood examinations. In all cases the rate of flow prescribed must be carefully maintained and accurate records of the fluid given by this and by any other route and of the patient's fluid output must be kept.

The same apparatus as that used for blood and plasma transfusions is suitable (see pp. 256–263) and the instruments required for cutting down on a vein and tying in a cannula should be provided. Where the treatment is to be continued for several days a fine polythene tube which can be passed through a needle into the superficial vein and thence into a deep vein is usually preferred to a metal cannula, as there is then less likelihood of irritation of the vein wall and clot formation.

BLOOD AND PLASMA TRANSFUSION

The usual indications for transfusion of blood or plasma are severe hæmorrhage, burns and shock. Transfusion with whole blood or with concentrated red cells is also often required in the treatment of anæmia. The standard transfusion fluids provided by the Blood Transfusion Services of the United Kingdom are:

(1) Whole blood.
(2) Concentrated suspension of red blood cells.
(3) Dried plasma or serum, with sterile pyrogen-free fluid for reconstitution.

There are several plasma substitutes, obtainable from commercial firms, which are widely used, for example a polysaccharide, dextran.

Blood Transfusion

Blood Groups

Blood transfusion is often a life-saving measure, but unless stringent precautions are taken it is fraught with great hazards. The concept of transfusing blood from a healthy individual into the veins of a patient dying of hæmorrhage is by no means new; many attempts were made to perfect a technique which would save life in such an emergency, but unfortunately these frequently resulted in the death of the patient. The greatest transfusion risk was overcome when the reason why donated blood could produce such disastrous results was discovered early in the present century. This discovery showed that every individual has substances in his blood which react against "foreign" proteins, including, in some cases, the proteins in the blood cells of another human being. The effect of these antibody substances is to cause agglutination, or clumping, of the red blood cells. Sometimes, however, the individual will produce no antibodies in response to foreign red cells entering his blood stream and in this case the blood of the donor is said to be compatible with that of the recipient; in other words both these individuals belong to the same blood group. Human blood is therefore classified according to the type of red cell present and the most important classifications of these substances are known as the ABO and the Rhesus (Rh) systems. Both donor and recipient must belong to the same ABO and Rh group. As a further check, since subgroups may also be present and because people acquire agglutinating bodies in addition to the "natural" antibodies, it is also necessary to carry out direct tests matching the recipient's blood against the blood to be donated.

ABO System. Human blood falls into one of four ABO categories, A, B, AB or O. Groups AB and B are comparatively rare amongst European populations, most of whom belong either to the A or the O group.

Group A. This group has A antigens in the red cells and anti-B antibodies in the plasma.

Group B.   This group has B antigens in the red cells and anti-A antibodies in the plasma.

Group AB. This group has both A and B antigens but the plasma contains no anti-A or B antibodies.

Group O.   This group has no A or B antigens in the red cells but has both anti-A and anti-B antibodies in the plasma.

Group A therefore cannot receive blood from Group B as the B group contains anti-A antibodies.

Group B similarly cannot receive from Group A.

Group AB has no anti-A or B antibodies and therefore, at least theoretically, can receive blood from all other groups.

Group O has both anti-A and anti-B antibodies and can therefore receive only Group O blood, but as Group O contains neither A nor B antibodies this group can give to all other ABO groups since the red cells of O group will not be agglutinated by the recipient's plasma. Group O is sometimes referred to as the "universal donor group" and may in cases of extreme emergency be given to a patient without awaiting the results of full cross-matching tests.

Rhesus Group System. The Rhesus, or Rh group, was given this name as it was found that the same system of antibodies was present in the blood of the rhesus monkey. In this system the most important factor is labelled "D"; the majority of Europeans have this D substance in their blood and are therefore described as Rh positive. About 15 per cent. of the population, however, do not have the Rh factor and are said to be Rh negative; transfusion of Rh positive blood to a Rh negative individual can be dangerous, since the Rh negative blood will produce antibodies to destroy the transfused cells. The effect of a first transfusion may be slight but the individual is liable to become sensitive to the D factor and further transfusions with Rh positive blood may produce a serious reaction. A similar reaction can take place in the blood of the fœtus in cases where the mother's blood is Rh negative but that of the fœtus is Rh positive. The maternal blood then produces antibodies which enter the fœtal circulation via the placenta and destroy the fœtal red blood cells. The fœtus may die or, if it survives to term, the infant may be born with a severe type of hæmolytic jaundice. Since sensitivity to the D factor takes some time to develop it is unusual for this reaction to occur in a first pregnancy. If a Rh negative girl or woman of child-bearing age is transfused with Rh positive blood this can also be the cause of a hæmolytic reaction should the woman become pregnant with a Rh positive fœtus, as her blood will in the meantime have produced Rh antibodies.

The bottles containing whole blood supplied by the Blood Transfusion Services are labelled to show the ABO and Rh groups, the date of collection of the blood from the donor and the date after which the blood is unfit for transfusion. Each bottle of stored whole blood contains 120 ml. of an anticoagulant solution, 1·66 per cent. disodium hydrogen citrate and 2·5 per cent. glucose. Stocks for hospital blood banks and sterilized, disposable, giving sets are supplied from regional centres of the Blood Transfusion Services. Mobile units from these centres also arrange donor sessions, at a hospital or other convenient place where blood is collected to maintain the stocks held at the regional centre. The "standard" type of donor set is being replaced by the disposable plastic set which is, however, not as yet universally available.

Requirements for Transfusion

Container with the blood or other fluid as prescribed.

Recipient set—a sterilized "disposable" nylon and polythene set which is used once and then discarded is now in general use. This set, which is illustrated in Fig. 21.2, consists of:

(1) A sterile intravenous needle with a Luer fitting in a glass container.

(2) Luer fitting mount attached to a short piece of rubber tubing (3) through which drugs can be injected intravenously, if necessary, while the transfusion is running. The proximal end of the rubber tubing is connected to a length of polythene tubing.

(4) Clamp for regulating the flow.

(5) Combined nylon filter and drop counter.

(6) Needle for piercing the bung of the container attached to delivery tube.

(7) Air inlet filter to be hooked above the fluid level in the container.

The piercing needle and air inlet tube are protected by plastic

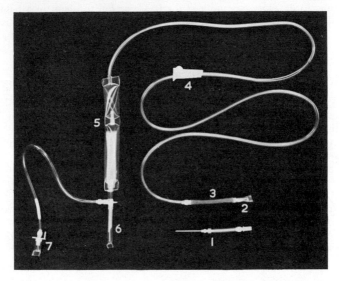

Fig. 21.2. DISPOSABLE POLYTHENE "GIVING" SET.

sheaths which must, of course, be removed when the apparatus is set up. Other requirements include:

A small sterile pack containing towels and swabs.

Cetrimide or other skin cleansing agent.

Sphygmomanometer to act as a torniquet to distend the superficial veins.

Adhesive strapping and scissors.

Instruments for cutting down on a vein and tying in a cannula:

(1) Scalpel or knife handle and blade.
(2) One pair of toothed fine dissecting forceps.
(3) One pair of non-toothed fine dissecting forceps.
(4) One pair of fine pointed scissors.
(5) Two fine artery forceps.
(6) Aneurysm needle.
(7) Thread size 60, or catgut size 00.

(8) Two curved skin needles and sutures.

(9) Intravenous cannula or fine polythene tubing with an adaptor.

(10) Hypodermic syringe, needle and local anæsthetic.

Setting up a Transfusion

When setting up the transfusion, or intravenous infusion, using the disposable recipient set the first step is to remove the protective sheath from the piercing needle of the delivery tube and to push the needle up to its flange into the bung of the container. The clamp on the delivery tube is closed, the container is suspended on the transfusion stand and the air inlet tube is hooked into position, making sure that the opening will be above the level of the fluid in the container. The drip chamber is filled by squeezing it once or twice, the protective sheath on the air inlet tube is removed, the tubing clamp is released to allow the fluid to run through the apparatus to expel air and is then closed. Meanwhile the skin at the site of the injection is cleaned, the sphygmomanometer cuff is placed round a limb, usually the arm, and blown up sufficiently to distend the veins while the doctor inserts the intravenous needle or ties in the cannula, whichever method is used. When the vein is entered the sphygmomanometer cuff is released and the needle or cannula connected to the Luer mount of the recipient set. The tubing clamp is adjusted to give the required rate of flow. The intravenous needle should be kept in position with adhesive strapping and the patient's arm or leg supported in a comfortable position. In the case of infants, young children, or very restless patients it may be found necessary to splint the limb. The strapping or bandage used to fix the splint must be taken over bony prominences in order to avoid the risk of obstructing the venous circulation. The veins of the scalp may be used in infants instead of the veins in the arm or leg.

Management of Transfusions

In all cases where a blood transfusion is likely to be needed 5 ml. of the patient's blood is obtained and sent to the laboratory for grouping and direct cross-matching tests with the sample of the blood to be transfused.

The correct blood for the individual patient is then labelled with his name, number and ward, and the statement that the blood is compatible is signed. The particulars on the label should

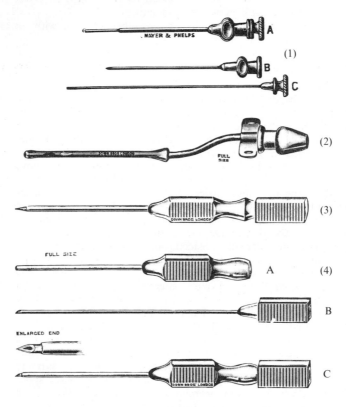

Fig. 21.3. VARIOUS TYPES OF INTRAVENOUS CANNULAE.

    (1) Bateman's Needle (for infants).
        A, Outer needle with stilette.
        B, Fine inner needle.
        C, Stilette.
    (2) Hamilton Bailey's gold-plated cannula.
    (3) Frankis Evans's intravenous needle.
    (4) West Middlesex Trocar and Cannula.
        A. Outer cannula.
        B. Trocar.
        C. Cannula and trocar fitted together.

be checked when the bottle or bottles are moved from the bank to the ward in order to ensure that the right blood is given to the right patient. Almost every case of incompatible transfusion is the result of an administrative error, *e.g.* incorrect labelling or failure to check the label carefully, particularly when there are two patients in the same ward with the same name.

Stored blood must be kept at a temperature between 4°C and 6°C (39°F to 43°F) in a thermostatically controlled refrigerator. It should never be cooled below 4°C or heated in any way. Bottles containing blood must always be carefully handled to avoid shaking the contents.

Whole blood may be used up to 21 days after withdrawal from the donor, provided that it is properly stored. Red cell suspensions, which are prepared by siphoning off the plasma from one or more bottles of whole blood and pooling the red cells, must be used within 24 hours of preparation.

Rate of Flow. Forty drops per minute is the usual rate for a slow transfusion. Rapid transfusion may be needed to replace a severe and sudden loss of blood and in such cases one or more bottles of blood may be given as rapidly as the blood will flow into the vein. In extreme urgency intra-arterial transfusion has been given, but is now little used.

Changing Bottles. A full bottle must be obtained from the bank and checked before the bottle in use is empty. The fresh bottle and a pair of sterile forceps are placed in a trolley at the bedside. When the blood level is just above the neck of the bottle in use the tubing clip above the drip chamber is closed; a second clamp may be applied as an extra safeguard against air entry. The bottle is unhooked and put on the trolley alongside the new bottle; the washer of this bottle is removed with the sterile forceps and the bung with the delivery and air inlet tubes is transferred from the old bottle. If a disposable container is used, all that is needed is to remove the piercing needle from the old bottle and insert it into the new bottle after removing the adhesive strip that protects the sterile bung. The needle must not be allowed to touch the edge or the outside of either bottle during this procedure. The full bottle is then suspended from the transfusion stand, the tubing clamp opened and the transfusion continued at the prescribed rate.

Difficulties that may arise during a Transfusion

Difficulty in maintaining the flow of blood may be due to one of several causes. The vein may go into spasm. This may be overcome by gently warming the limb or by stroking along the vein above the injection site.

The tubing may become kinked or pressed upon and this possibility should always be borne in mind and careful inspection made.

The needle may become dislodged. An attempt may be made to alter the position of needle by gently lifting the mount to depress the point. This may be successful, but if the needle has punctured the wall of the vein the transfusion will have to be stopped and if necessary started again using another vein.

An air-lock may block the flow of blood from the bottle. This should not occur if due care is taken to expel all air from the delivery tubing before connecting it to the needle or cannula. If, however, an air-lock should be present the apparatus must be disconnected from the needle and blood allowed to run freely through the tubing before it is again connected to the intravenous needle.

The introduction of large volumes of blood, or any other fluid, into the blood-stream can give rise to cardiac and respiratory distress as a result of overloading the circulatory system. This danger is greatest when large quantities of fluid are rapidly introduced, but can occur with a slow transfusion particularly in elderly patients with a weakened heart muscle or chronic anæmia. Signs which should be watched for and reported to the medical officer immediately are: rising pulse rate, laboured breathing, cough, pain in the chest and œdema. A fluid intake and output chart should always be kept for a patient who is receiving parenteral fluid.

A severe reaction occurring soon after the transfusion has been started may be due to incompatibility of the blood and hæmolysis of the red cells. The symptoms are: shivering and rise of temperature, the patient may complain of severe pain in the lumbar region. The transfusion must be stopped at once. There is great danger of renal failure due to the blocking of the renal tubules by hæmolysed blood cells with subsequent suppression of urine and uræmia.

Pyrexial reaction due to the introduction of foreign protein into the blood can also give rise to rigors, fever and an increased pulse rate. The rate of the transfusion should be slowed, or the transfusion may have to be stopped.

Thrombosis of the vein is not uncommon. It may be limited in extent and cause little trouble, but if extensive there is considerable pain in the limb and there may be a rise in the patient's temperature. The transfusion may have to be discontinued and a hot application may be ordered for the relief of pain.

A hæmatoma may form at the site of the transfusion, this results from the needle becoming dislodged from the vein and the blood is then extravasated into the surrounding tissues. The transfusion must be stopped and the limb elevated. An injection of Hyalase may be given into the swollen area. There is some danger when the swelling occurs on the anterior aspect of the forearm and elbow that the arteries supplying the forearm may be compressed and careful watch should be kept on the radial pulse and also on the fingers for blueness and coldness.

Sepsis may occur at the site of the infusion. This is more liable to occur when a cannula is tied into the vein than with the use of an intravenous needle.

Air embolism is a rare occurrence but one which must be borne in mind. It is prevented by making sure that air is entirely expelled from the tubing before the transfusion is started, by taking care that the bottle is not allowed to run dry, and by seeing that the arm into which the transfusion is running is never raised above the level of the patient's heart as this can cause air to be sucked into the vein if the bottle is empty. If it is necessary to increase the rate of flow this can be done by raising the level of the bottle; pressure should never be used to make the blood run faster. The patient may complain of a variety of sensory disturbances, *e.g.* tingling in the fingers, and may collapse. The immediate treatment is to lower the patient's head.

Transfusion of Plasma and Plasma Substitutes

Dried blood plasma can be stored for long periods without deterioration and can be reconstituted with the pyrogen-free fluid supplied by the Blood Transfusion Services when required. Plasma transfusions are often given in the treatment of shock and in cases where large amounts of plasma have been lost, as in extensive burning. In an emergency plasma can be used in place of blood while awaiting the results of cross-matching tests. The main risk in the use of plasma is the possibility of transmitting a virus disease, homologous hepatitis.

Plasma is expensive and various substitutes are available which have the same osmotic pressure and the necessary viscosity and molecular weight to enable them to act as "plasma expanders"; examples of these are dextran and Dextraven. Plasma substitutes are free from the risk of transmitting virus infection.

22 THE ADMINISTRATION OF ENEMAS: RECTAL LAVAGE: ABDOMINAL AND RECTAL EXAMINATIONS

Enemas

An enema is an injection of fluid into the rectum and this may be ordered for various reasons:
(1) To empty the bowel of fæces.
(2) To introduce drugs or fluids.
(3) For diagnostic purposes.

Apparatus. For large quantities such as are used for cleansing the bowel, a douche can, a piece of tubing about 24 inches long, a connector and also a rectal tube or catheter, size 14 or 16, are required. A Higginson's syringe with a rectal tube attached is occasionally used and in this case the solution to be injected is placed in a bowl. For small quantities a glass funnel or the barrel of a glass syringe is connected to a rubber catheter (size 8). The same apparatus is usually used for giving an enema to a child.

Important Points to be observed in giving an Enema. The rectum is not a straight tube, it curves backwards, following the contour of the coccyx and the sacrum. The rectal tube should be passed first forward and upward, through the anal canal, which is approximately two inches in length, into the lower end of the rectum.

The flow of the fluid will be helped if the patient lies on her left side, or, if on her back, has the pelvis raised during the administration of the enema. The douche can should be raised about 12 inches above the level of the patient's body.

The length of the rectum is about 6 inches, and if more than 4 to 6 inches of the tube is passed it is liable to kink or to become coiled upon itself. This is uncomfortable for the patient and also obstructs the flow of the enema fluid.

No force should be used in passing a rectal tube. If the anal sphincter is tightly closed or the patient has hæmorrhoids, which make the part very sensitive, it may be necessary to dilate the sphincter before passing the tube, using the finger protected by a rubber glove or finger stall lubricated with petroleum jelly. The tube should be well lubricated and air expelled by allowing the fluid to run through, before inserting it.

The tube should be inserted about 4 inches into the rectum, so that it is well gripped by the anal sphincter, and a brief pause should follow the insertion before allowing the fluid to flow. To ensure that the fluid flows right round to the cæcum, when this is required for cleansing or for treatment, it should not be injected too quickly and the pelvis should be raised (if this is not possible, the foot of the bed may be raised).

The enema must be given at the right temperature, usually 37·5°–40°C (100°–105°F).

A report of the result of the enema should always be made, and, if necessary the result saved for inspection. If obstruction is suspected it is important to note the passage of flatus.

The procedure should always be simply explained to the patient before beginning the treatment. A very ill patient or a patient who has been given an enema for the relief of distension, when it is important to note if flatus is passed, should not be left until the bed-pan has been removed.

It is usual to protect the bed with a warmed mackintosh, which may be covered with a cotton square or a piece of cellulose. After giving the enema, the rectal catheter should be disconnected and placed in a receiver so that it does not soil anything else. It should be flushed through with cold water, washed well with warm soapy water to remove the grease and boiled for five minutes.

Complications that may result from giving an enema are:

(1) Faintness and collapse, due to the distension of the rectum with fluid.

(2) An enema rash. If the patient states that on a previous occasion a rash followed the giving of a soap enema, this should be reported.

(3) Possible perforation of the rectal wall if a rigid nozzle is used.

Cleansing Enemas

Water. A suitable quantity of warm water injected into the bowel will distend the rectum, wash out the lower bowel and produce an evacuant action. Water is as effective and less irritating than the traditional soap and water enema. The quantity required will vary from a few ounces for a young child to 1 to 3 pints for an adult.

Soap and Water. From 1 to 3 pints of the solution will be required for an adult.

A soap solution ready made up is often used in hospital, and the enema is prepared by adding the directed quantity of the soap solution to hot water. Green soft soap one ounce to one pint of water may be used, and a piece about the size of a large walnut will be required for every pint of water. The soap should be well beaten into the water and the solution strained before use.

Recently attention has been drawn to the fact that the injection of large quantities of water or of soap and water into the bowel can be a dangerous process as these fluids are rapidly absorbed from the colon into the blood stream and may bring about a serious change in the concentration of electrolytes in the blood. The symptoms produced are due to what is known as "water intoxication" and include nausea, vomiting and drowsiness which may proceed to a state of coma and convulsions; the patient's breathing may become rapid and irregular. The danger is greatest in young children and when repeated enemas are given. It is important that the nurse should be aware of this danger and that she should appreciate the importance of accurate measurement of the fluid injected and the fluid returned when administering enemas or any form of bowel wash-out. The sodium phosphate enema described below is considerably safer from this point of view in that only a small quantity of fluid is injected.

Sodium Phosphate. Recently the use of mixed sodium phosphates dissolved in a small quantity of water as an evacuant enema has been adopted in hospital practice and in home nursing. A solution of sodium dihydrogen phosphate 14 grammes and disodium hydrogen phosphate 4 grammes in 120 ml. of water is equally, if not more effective than a soap and water enema and causes the patient less discomfort. Disposable plastic units with a plastic or rubber injection tube are available. The administration of the enema is simple and the apparatus is used once only so that the task of cleaning and boiling equipment after use is eliminated.

Olive Oil. Warm olive oil may be ordered to soften the fæces after operations on the rectum or perineum (when it is necessary to ensure that no hard masses be passed), or in cases of impacted fæces; 4 to 10 fl. oz. of warm olive oil is slowly injected with a catheter and funnel. The patient should retain this for at least half an hour, and the treatment is completed by giving a soap-and-water enema if ordered.

Enemas used to Introduce Drugs for their General or Local Effect

Magnesium Sulphate Enema. Magnesium sulphate solution given as an enema attracts fluid from the tissues into the bowel. It may be ordered as an evacuant and also in cases of raised intracranial tension in order to relieve the tension by causing dehydration of the tissues. For this purpose 6 to 8 fl. oz. of a 50 per cent. solution of magnesium sulphate may be given twice a day for several days.

Starch and Opium Enema. A starch mucilage usually with the addition of tincture of opium may be ordered for the relief of diarrhœa. A starch and opium enema consists of 15 to 30 minims of tincture of opium as ordered, 2 to 4 oz. of starch mucilage.

1 oz. of the starch mucilage should be injected slowly at body temperature, using a No. 8 catheter and a small funnel or barrel of a glass syringe, then the ordered amount of opium is given, followed by a sufficient amount of the mucilage to clear the opium from the funnel and tubing.

To make the mucilage take a dessertspoonful of powdered starch and sufficient cold water to make a stiff paste. Add sufficient boiling water to make a fluid which will be thin enough to run through the enema apparatus when cooled to 35·7°C (100°F).

An alternative method is to take 1 level dessertspoonful of starch, mixing this to a smooth thin paste with 5 oz. of cold water. The mixture is brought to the boil and boiled for 2 minutes. One teaspoonful of cold water is added and the mucilage is allowed to cool.

Cortisone Enema. Hydrocortisone in normal saline may be ordered as a retention enema in the treatment of ulcerative colitis. 100 mg. of hydrocortisone hemi-succinate is mixed with about 120 ml. of normal saline. The enema is given at body heat using a rubber catheter and a small funnel. The administration should take 20 to 30 minutes.

Diagnostic Enema

The barium sulphate emulsion for use in barium enema X-ray examinations is usually made up in the dispensary in the form of a barium suspension.

The following prescription is one in use:

Barium sulphate	..	..	..	..	.. 40 oz.
Tragacanth powder		..	..	..	60 grains
Water	..	..	..	..	To 80 fluid oz.

This is to be diluted with an equal quantity of water for use. The water added to the emulsion should be hot enough to bring the mixture to body temperature.

The colon and rectum should be empty before the barium enema is administered, an aperient is usually ordered twenty-four hours before hand and a rectal wash-out given about four hours before the X-ray examination. The preparation used in some diagnostic X-ray departments may vary from that described and exact instructions should always be obtained.

Retention Enemas as a Means of administering Fluid

Rectal administration of normal saline solution or of water is a method of supplementing the fluid intake. 5 or 10 per cent. glucose may be added.

If the patient is to retain and absorb the fluid satisfactorily the following points must receive attention:

(1) The rectum and the bladder must be empty.

(2) The fluid must be injected slowly.

Method 1. The required amount of tap water or saline and glucose solution, usually not more than 10 oz., is run in slowly, using a No. 8 rubber catheter and a small funnel or the barrel of a glass syringe.

In order to have complete control over the rate of flow the funnel should be held at a level only slightly above that of the patient's body. The rate of flow must be slow and even.

10 oz. of fluid should take at least ten minutes to give. The patient should be left undisturbed for half an hour after the injection.

This method may also be used for the injection of basal anæsthetics or narcotics such as paraldehyde and bromethol.

Method 2 ("*Continuous Drip*"). A glass bottle is required, fitted with a rubber bung with two holes.

A short glass tube fixed in one hole is connected to a piece of

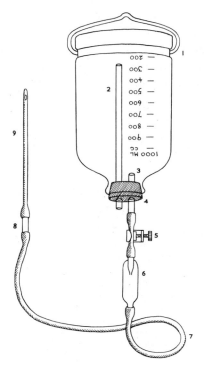

Fig. 22.1. APPARATUS FOR "CONTINUOUS DRIP" RECTAL SALINE INFUSION.

    (1) Metal band and handle for suspension.
    (2) Metal tube acting as an air inlet.
    (3) Metal outlet tube.
    (4) Black rubber bung.
    (5) Short piece of rubber tubing and screw clip.
    (6) Drop counter.
    (7) Length of rubber tubing.
    (8) Connector.
    (9) Rubber catheter.

rubber tubing with a screw-clip. A further piece of rubber tubing, a connector and a No. 7 or 8 rubber catheter are required.

A second glass tube long enough to reach to the far end of the bottle passes through the second hole in the bung, this acts as an airway.

The fluid is allowed to run through the tubing to expel the air, and the tubing is then clipped and the container suspended at the bedside neck downwards. The tubing clip is regulated to give the required rate of flow (about 1 drop per second). Several pints of fluid may be slowly introduced by this method.

The nurse should see that the steady rate of flow is maintained and should also make sure from time to time that the patient is retaining the fluid.

Rectal Suppositories

Rectal suppositories are now often ordered in place of enemas and rectal wash-outs in the preparation of the patient for various examinations, such as X-ray examinations of the intestinal and renal tracts. Bisacodyl (Dulcolax) suppositories, in conjunction with Dulcolax tablets by mouth, are usually effective. This form of preparation can be self-administered and is therefore particularly convenient for out-patients.

Glycerin suppositories are available in sizes suitable for children and for adults and may be useful in softening hard fæces in the rectum and producing an action of the bowels with little disturbance of the patient.

Passing a Flatus Tube for the Relief of Distension

Requirements:

(1) A rubber rectal tube. This tube has thick walls and the eye is at the end. (In this respect it differs from a catheter which has a lateral eye.) A connector attaching the rectal tube to a length of tubing with a funnel at the other end.

(2) Petroleum jelly, or other lubricant and swabs.

(3) A bowl of water.

(4) A receiver for soiled swabs.

(5) A mackintosh square and pad to protect the bed.

The tube is lubricated and passed into the rectum to a depth of about 2 inches. The funnel is placed under the surface of the water in the bowl which is placed at the bedside. The advantage of attaching the tube to a funnel placed in a bowl of water is that the bubbles of gas can be readily seen as they escape from the funnel.

Rectal and Colonic Lavage

This treatment may be ordered in the preparation of a patient for examination by sigmoidoscopy or for a barium enema examination.

Requirements:

A rubber catheter, size 14, or rectal tube.

A length of rubber tubing.

A tubing clip.

A connector to fit the rubber tubing and the catheter.

Lubricant and swabs.

A large jug containing the washout fluid, usually water or normal saline. Six pints or more may be needed.

An irrigating can, or a large funnel and a pint measure jug.

A pail to receive returned fluid or a large bed-pan.

Receiver for soiled swabs and catheter.

The water or lotion should be prepared at a temperature of 40°C (105°F) and used at a temperature of 37·5°C (100°F).

The catheter is lubricated, fluid is poured into the irrigating can and allowed to run through the apparatus to expel air and the tubing is then clamped with the tubing clip. If a funnel is used in place of the irrigating can it is filled from the pint measure jug.

The patient lies on his left side with the knees flexed and the catheter is passed into the rectum for a distance of about three inches. The clip is released and fluid allowed to flow, it should run in slowly at first as sudden distension of the rectum may cause the patient to return the fluid. When one pint has been given the patient should, if possible, turn into the "knee-chest" position while a further pint is allowed to run in steadily, then he assumes the right lateral position while the third pint is given. The tubing is then clipped, the catheter removed and the patient placed on the bed-pan and allowed to return the wash-out fluid.

An alternative method is to run in about half a pint of fluid using a large funnel and then to siphon it back by inverting the funnel over a pail. The process is repeated until the fluid returns clear.

Accurate measurement of the fluid given and the fluid returned must always be made.

Abdominal Examination

The bed should be screened and nearby windows closed. The patient should lie on her back with the knees slightly flexed and one pillow under the head and shoulders. The bedclothes should be turned down to the thighs and the patient left covered with the sheet. The nightgown should be folded up to the breasts and a small blanket or shawl arranged to cover the chest. When the doctor is ready to make the examination the nurse should turn down the sheet and arrange the chest blanket so that the area from the breasts to the pubes is bare. During the examination the nurse should stand at the left-hand side of the bed at the head end. Requirements for rectal examination should be at hand.

Rectal Examination

Requirements:

A right-hand rubber or disposable polythene glove or caped finger stall.

Glove powder.

Lubricant.

Swabs.

Receiver.

A rectal speculum and a hand lamp may be needed.

The patient should, if possible, lie in the left lateral position with the buttocks brought to the edge of the bed and the knees flexed.

The gown should be folded up over the chest; a blanket is arranged to cover the chest and the buttocks are covered by a sheet only. During the examination the nurse should stand at the right-hand side of the bed.

Examination by Sigmoidoscopy

This examination is carried out in the theatre. It is important that the rectum should be emptied of fæces and also of any fluid given as an enema or rectal wash-out.

The actual preparation will vary according to the wish of the surgeon, but the following may be taken as a guide:

Thirty-six hours before the examination the patient is given an aperient.

Twelve hours before the examination the patient is given a soap-and-water enema or a rectal wash-out with plain warm water. The nurse should measure all fluid injected and the fluid returned. Should fluid be left behind in the bowel, the examination is likely to be a failure because it would obscure the view through the sigmoidoscope.

Following this preparation a dose of tincture of opium may be ordered to allay further bowel movement.

23 CATHETERIZATION, IRRIGATION AND DRAINAGE OF THE URINARY BLADDER

Catheterization

Catheterization of the urinary bladder may be required to relieve distension of the bladder when the patient is unable to pass urine, to empty the bladder before an operation on the pelvic organs or to obtain a specimen of urine for examination.

Varieties of Catheters

Soft Rubber. These are in sizes from 1 to 20, English gauge. The size most often required for catheterization is 8.

Elastic Gum. In the same sizes as the rubber catheters. French catheters, however, are numbered from 1 to 30. The elastic gum catheter may be straight with a bulbous or cylindrical end, or may be angled or "elbowed" near the eye. In the latter case it is known as a coudé catheter. If it has two bends it is a bicoudé catheter.

Plastic materials: such as polyvinyl.

Metal Catheters. These are made in both the male and female patterns. Metal female catheters may be used in midwifery practice.

Catheterization of a Male Patient

The doctor may select the catheters, but if there are no special orders the nurse should sterilize rubber and elastic gum catheters, sizes 7 and 8. Polyvinyl catheters may be supplied ready for use in individual sterile packs.

Requirements:

Sterile catheters in a sterile tray dry or in cold sterile water, or normal saline solution.

A lubricant, such as sterile glycerin or liquid paraffin.

Sterile towels and swabs.

Bowl of warm lotion for swabbing, *e.g.* Hibitane 0·1 per cent., Bradosol 1 in 2,000 solution.

Large receiver for urine.

Mackintosh.

Receiver for dirty swabs.

(If a "clean" specimen for examination is required, a sterile screw-top bottle to receive the urine must be provided.)

The bed is screened and the bedclothes arranged so that they can be easily turned down over the thighs, leaving the abdomen and chest covered with a blanket.

After the trolley is brought to the bedside the nurse is not usually required to give any further assistance.

If the catheter is to be tied in, the following should also be provided:

Tape.

Adhesive strapping.

A pair of scissors.

If urethral bougies are to be passed these are sterilized in the same way as catheters. The same trolley should be set as for catheterization.

Catheterization of a Female Patient

Requirements:

Two sterilized catheters in a sterile bowl or dish.

A bowl of lotion for swabbing.

Sterile swabs and towels.

Mackintosh.

Large receiver for urine.

Receiver for dirty swabs.

A hand lamp.

A lubricant is not as a rule required.

(When a sterile specimen is required a sterile screw-top bottle should be provided, and all traces of antiseptics should be removed by swabbing with sterile water.)

The bed should be screened and the bedclothes turned down from the patient's knees, leaving her covered with a blanket. A warmed mackintosh is placed under the patient's thighs and buttocks and a receiver or a porringer between her legs. The hand lamp should be adjusted so that it gives a good light; it is absolutely essential that the nurse should be able to obtain a clear view of the area when swabbing the external genitals and when actually passing the catheter.

The nurse then prepares her hands by washing and drying them on a clean towel. When she returns to the bedside she turns back the covering blanket with her elbow, or asks an assistant to do this for her.

Using swabs well moistened with the antiseptic lotion she swabs the external genital region beginning with the labia majora, then swabbing the labia minora and lastly the area around the urethral orifice. Each swab should be used once only and the direction of swabbing should be from the anterior aspect of the vulva towards the posterior margin. The nurse should then wash her hands once more and arrange the sterile towels to cover the patient's thighs. The catheter should be picked up in the right hand, the first finger and thumb of the left hand being used to separate the labia. The urethral orifice should be clearly seen and a good light is essential, the opening is situated immediately in front of the vaginal orifice and at the base of the triangular area known as the vestibule. A metal or plastic catheter may be held sufficiently far from the tip to ensure that the section handled does not enter the urethra, this is more difficult with a soft rubber catheter and sterile forceps or piece of sterile gauze may be used to avoid direct handling of the catheter. The tip of the catheter is passed into the urethral orifice and then the instrument is pushed on in an upward and backward direction for about two inches, leaving the open end in the receiver between the patient's thighs. If the catheter should accidentally touch any adjacent part before it is safely inserted in the urethra it should be discarded as probably contaminated and the second sterile catheter should then be used.

If a catheter specimen is required for laboratory examination it is collected in a sterile screw-top glass bottle.

When urine ceases to flow the nurse should make gentle pressure over the pubes and withdraw the catheter for about half an inch, when she feels sure that the bladder is empty the catheter is withdrawn and placed in the receiver provided. The porringer is removed, the vulva dried and the bed remade. The amount of urine withdrawn should be measured and a specimen saved if required.

Catheterization is a procedure that should be carried out with the utmost care with regard to the sterilization of the catheters, the cleansing of the vulva beforehand and the skilful manipulation of the catheter. Infection of the urinary tract can occur very readily and may be very serious. Patients who are being regularly catheterized may be given one of the chemotherapeutic drugs, such as Furadantin. Frequent catheterization is avoided whenever possible in neurological cases; where incontinence occurs Paul's tubing may be secured to the penis to avoid the necessity.

Irrigation of the Bladder

Irrigation of the bladder is seldom used except in conjunction with drainage by an in-dwelling catheter (as in "tidal drainage") or in male patients following a genito-urinary operation, such as prostatectomy or lithotomy, when it may be necessary to wash out blood and debris. A metal bladder syringe is used or a funnel with a length of tubing to attach it to the in-dwelling catheter. Normal saline solution or sterile water may be used for the wash out.

Bladder Drainage

Continuous or Intermittent Drainage with an In-dwelling Catheter. Drainage of the bladder with an in-dwelling catheter is often needed for paraplegic patients with urinary incontinence. Retention of urine with overflow is a common feature of this condition and leads to the complication of urinary stasis and infection.

In male patients Gibbon's fine (4 to 12 French gauge) polyvinyl catheter is often used. It is less irritating to the urethra than a rubber catheter and can be left in position for an indefinite time, usually until it becomes blocked with mucus or deposits. The Gibbon catheter is 5 feet long with a rounded end and three side holes; 12 inches from the tip two soft wings are attached so that it can be secured to the abdominal wall (Fig. 23.1).

These catheters can be boiled or sterilized in the autoclave and are introduced with full aseptic precautions. The pubic area is washed and shaved and the skin of the area and the penis is cleaned with an antiseptic, such as Hibitane 0·1 per cent. The procedure may be carried out in the theatre. The free end of the catheter drains into a sterile receptacle attached to the patient's

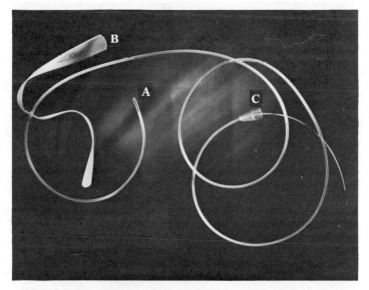

Fig. 23.1. POLYVINYL GIBBON'S IN-DWELLING CATHETER.

A. Tip of Catheter with three side holes.
B. Wings of soft material cemented 12 inches from lip which are strapped to the patient's abdomen.
C. Graduated adapter which fits the tube of the collecting bag or bottle.

bed. A "Portex" urine collecting and measuring bag (Fig. 23.2) is very suitable for this purpose.

Various modifications of the original Gibbon catheter have been produced. Some authorities prefer a larger gauge catheter such as size 18 (French gauge). The fine tubing of the Gibbon catheter tends to slip out of the female urethra and either a size 18 Gibbon type or Foley's self-retaining catheter (Fig. 23.3) is more suitable for female patients.

Intermittent drainage may be used to encourage the development of periodic, automatic emptying of the bladder. In this case a sterile spigot is kept in the end of the catheter and released at intervals, usually every three hours.

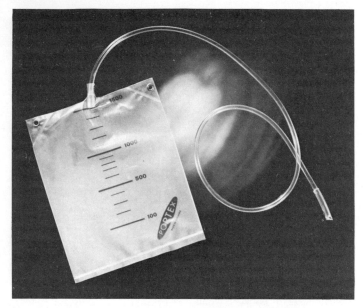

Fig. 23.2. DISPOSABLE URINE COLLECTING AND MEASURING BAG FOR USE WITH GIBBON'S OR OTHER TYPES OF IN-DWELLING CATHETERS.

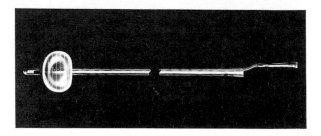

Fig. 23.3. FOLEY'S URETHRAL CATHETER.

Tidal Drainage

This combination of drainage and irrigation may be used in cases of residual infection in the bladder. A large receptacle for the irrigating lotion is connected to a drip outlet which in turn is joined by a piece of rubber tubing to one arm of a Y-shaped glass

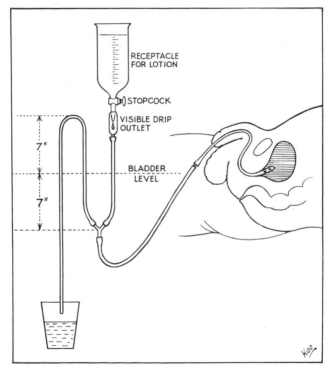

RECEPTACLE FOR LOTION

STOPCOCK

VISIBLE DRIP OUTLET

BLADDER LEVEL

7"

7"

Fig. 23.4. TIDAL DRAINAGE.

connection (Fig. 23.4). The stem of this connection is attached to a catheter in the patient's bladder, the remaining arm to a length of rubber tubing which is looped to form a U-shaped manometer fourteen inches high with the centre at the level of the patient's bladder. The end of this long piece of tubing opens into a pail on the floor which collects the fluid. The lotion is allowed to drip slowly into the bladder via the catheter; as the bladder fills with the lotion and with urine the pressure in the U loop rises, and when the fluid reaches the top of the U it empties by siphonage into the pail. The bladder then begins to fill again.

24 VAGINAL EXAMINATION AND IRRIGATION: VULVAL TOILET: VAGINAL PESSARIES

Vaginal Examination

A vaginal examination may be required in order to determine the position of the uterus, the presence and position of a pelvic mass, for inspection of the vagina and cervix uteri, or to obtain material for pathological investigations.

In the ward, or clinic, the examination is usually carried out with a speculum and the surgeon's gloved hand. More extensive examinations, often including a cervical smear or biopsy, are carried out under general anæsthesia in the theatre.

For a simple examination no preparation of the patient is usually required; an aperient may be given on the day before the examination if it is needed. Out-patients should be instructed to remove all top clothing, corsets and knickers and to come to the examination couch wearing a vest or loose slip, stockings, slippers and a dressing gown.

The patient is usually examined in the dorsal (Fig. 24A) and the left lateral positions (Fig. 24B). Other "gynæcological" positions which may be used are:

Semi-lateral or Sims's Position. The patient lies on her left side with the buttocks brought to the side of the bed and the upper leg rather more flexed than the under one. The head and chest should lie prone on the bed with one small pillow. The left arm hangs over the edge of the bed and the right arm is brought up alongside the pillow (Fig. 24C).

The Upright Position. The patient stands at the side of a chair with one foot resting on the rung and steadying herself with one hand on the back of the chair. This position is sometimes required when an examination is made for prolapse.

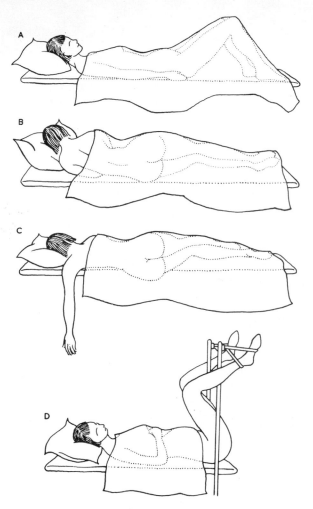

Fig. 24.1. GYNAECOLOGICAL POSITIONS.
   A. Dorsal position.
   B. Left lateral position.
   C. Semi-lateral or Sims's position.
   D. Lithotomy position.

Lithotomy Position. The patient lies on her back with the knees flexed and the thighs raised and separated. The buttocks are brought to the edge of the couch, the legs are supported in stirrups and the foot end of the examination couch is dropped (Fig. 24D).

Requirements for vaginal examination:

Right-hand rubber or "disposable" polythene gloves.

Receptacles for soiled swabs and for used instruments.

A bowl of lotion, *e.g.* Hibitane 0·1 per cent. Cetrimide 1 per cent. solution.

Swabs.

Swab-holding forceps.

Vaginal specula: Sims's duckbill, Ferguson's or bivalve type.

If a smear of discharge from the cervix is required the following should be prepared:

Ferguson's speculum.

Vulsellum forceps.

Swabs and a swab-holder.

A platinum wire loop, or sterile throat swabs.

Microscope slides.

A spirit lamp.

Labels.

Requirements for rectal examination should be provided.

Vaginal Irrigation (Douching)

Vaginal irrigation is usually ordered for cleansing purposes, *e.g.* before gynæcological operations, for patients wearing vaginal pessaries or for patients who have a vaginal discharge.

Hot douching at a temperature of 46° to 49°C (115° to 120°F) was at one time occasionally ordered for the arrest of uterine hæmorrhage or for the treatment of pelvic inflammation, but in the former case it is seldom effective and in the latter case chemotherapeutic drugs have replaced local treatment.

Requirements:

An irrigation can, three pint capacity (or 2 litres).

A long piece of tubing to fit the outlet of the can and the irrigation nozzle.

Soft rubber catheter or irrigation nozzle, which may be glass, rubber or plastic.

Tubing clip.

Jug containing the lotion as ordered; lotion thermometer.
Bowl with lotion for swabbing, *e.g.* Hibitane 0·1 per cent.
Sterile swabs and pads.
"Douche" pan or large "perfection" type bed-pan.
Receptacles for soiled swabs and for the soiled nozzle.

The apparatus may be sterilized by boiling and is then placed in a large sterile bowl. The lotion is prepared at a temperature of 40°C (105°F). As a general rule only mild lotions are used for cleansing, *e.g.* normal saline solution, 1 per cent. lactic acid or domiphen bromide (Bradosol) 1 in 2,000 solution.

The lotion is poured into the irrigating can and the tubing is clipped. The can should be hung about a foot above the level of the patient's pelvis so that the fluid will run in gently at low pressure.

The douche pan or bed-pan is placed under the patient, who should lie on her back with one or two pillows under the head and shoulders. A square of waterproof material can be used to protect the bottom sheet.

Before the nurse washes her hands the bedclothes should be so arranged that the patient's thighs and legs are covered by a blanket and sheet while her chest and abdomen are covered by a folded blanket. When the nurse returns from washing her hands and drying them on a clean towel, she pushes the lower half of the divided bedclothes down using her elbow. Taking a swab in her right hand she first swabs the labia majora with the antiseptic lotion provided and then parting the labia with the first finger and thumb of her left hand she swabs the labia minora and the area of the vaginal orifice. The swabbing should be carried out from above downwards and each swab should be used once only. The tubing clip is released allowing the lotion to flow through the apparatus. The nozzle or catheter is then inserted gently upwards and backwards into the vagina for about 3 inches.

When the irrigation is completed the patient should sit up on the douche pan for a few moments to allow the fluid to drain out of the vagina. The vulva is then dried with sterile swabs and a sterile pad applied.

A glass douche nozzle should always be carefully inspected before use to make sure that it is not cracked or chipped. In all cases where stitches have been inserted into the perineum or vagina it is safer to use a rubber catheter.

Vulval Toilet

In obstetric cases and in cases where the vulval or perineal area has been sutured, careful vulval toilet is necessary for the comfort of the patient and also in order to prevent infection of the sutured area. "Jug" douching may be ordered to cleanse the external genitalia and perineal area.

Vulval Swabbing and Dressing of Sutures

Requirements:

Sterile kidney dish.

Sterile bowl containing warm antiseptic lotion such as domiphen bromide (Bradosol) 1 in 2,000 solution or plain water.

Sterile bowl containing sterile swabs, gauze vulval pads, two
   pairs of dressing forceps.

Receptacle for soiled swabs and dressings.

First of all the patient's groins and the inner aspect of the thighs should be washed with soap and water and dried. The nurse should then wash and dry her hands. Taking a well moistened swab in her left hand she swabs the external aspect of the labia then, discarding that swab, she parts the labia with her left hand and with her right hand swabs the inner aspect of each labium, using one swab for each side. Next the area of the vestibule and the vaginal orifice is swabbed. The area should then be carefully dried and the vulval pad applied. The patient is then asked to bring her thighs together and to turn on her side. The vulval pad is folded back exposing the perineal area.

The suture area is dried with a sterile swab held in forceps and the antiseptic paint or powder is applied. The sutures are then covered with gauze, taking care to wrap the long ends of the sutures in the gauze so that they do not catch in the vulval pad when the patient moves. The vulval pad is brought down to cover the dressing and the pad is kept in place with a T bandage.

"Jug" Douching

For this procedure a two-pint jug containing warm antiseptic lotion or warm water and a large receiver or douche pan will be required, in addition to the items listed above.

Some of the lotion is first poured over the vulva and then the nurse separates the labia with her left hand and continues pouring the remainder of the lotion so that the flow of antiseptic cleanses the labia minora and vaginal orifice. On completion of the douching, the area is carefully dried with swabs and sterile vulval pad applied. If sutures have to be dressed the patient now turns on her side and this procedure is carried out as described above.

Vaginal Pessaries

A pessary is an instrument introduced into the vagina usually in order to afford support in the case of a prolapsed uterus. Pessaries are made of vulcanite, Perspex or coils of watch spring covered with rubber. Pessaries used in the treatment of uterine prolapse may be ring shaped or, if the vaginal walls and perineum are too lax to allow the ring to remain in position a circular cup with a stem, Napier's pessary, is inserted. The cup supports the cervix and the stem is attached by four tapes to a band round the patient's waist. The use of pessaries in the treatment of genital prolapse is now comparatively rare, since the majority of patients can be far more satisfactorily treated by operative measures. The nurse may be required to change a ring pessary.

Insertion of a Ring Pessary

Requirements:
Sterilized introducer or clip forceps and a length of tape.
Sterilized pessary, vulcanite, watch spring or Perspex.
Swabs in lotion, *e.g.* Bradosol 1 in 2,000 solution.
Sterile lubricant.
Sterile gloves.
Mackintosh.
Receptacle for soiled swabs.
Receiver for discarded gloves.
A good light is essential and an adjustable standard or hand
    lamp may be needed.

The patient is placed in the left lateral position and a mackintosh is arranged to protect the bed or couch. Before the pessary is inserted the nurse should swab the vulva and then after washing her hands again puts on the sterilized gloves. Taking the pessary in her right hand she dips it in the lubricant. The nurse's left hand is used to separate the labia. The ring is then inserted into the vagina with the posterior rim along the length of the orifice gradually turning it over directing it upwards and backwards until one side of the rim of the ring is in the posterior fornix and the cervix can be felt in the centre of the ring. The anterior rim is then pushed up above the symphysis pubis. If the watch spring pessary is used it is compressed into an elliptical shape and held in an introducer or by tying a piece of tape round it and clipping the tape with a pair of forceps. When the pessary has been introduced the forceps are released and the tape removed.

All patients who are wearing pessaries other than the Perspex type should have a daily vaginal douche and may be taught to carry out this treatment themselves. Patients should also be given instructions as to when they should see their doctor for changing or removing the pessary. A rubber pessary may need changing every six weeks, a vulcanite pessary may be left for three months. Any patient who experiences pain or discomfort should be advised to report to her doctor as soon as possible.

25 EXAMINATION AND TREATMENT OF THE EAR, THROAT, NOSE AND EYE: NEUROLOGICAL EXAMINATION

Examination of the Ear

Requirements:

Forehead mirror and lamp, or illuminating headlight.

Aural specula of various sizes.

Angular aural forceps.

Probes, *e.g.* Jobson-Horne ring probes.

Dressed wooden applicators.

Small wool swabs.

Receptacle for soiled swabs.

The patient should sit sideways with the ear to be examined opposite the doctor. If a forehead mirror is used the light from the lamp is directed so that it shines on the mirror.

If the auditory meatus is full of wax, the doctor will order the ear to be syringed before the examination can be completed.

To Syringe an Ear

Requirements:

An aural syringe. A metal syringe may be used, or a Higginson's bulb syringe with a straight Eustachian catheter attached.

Lotion, *e.g.* sodium chloride 0·9 per cent. (normal saline) or sodium bicarbonate, 1 teaspoonful to water 1 pint.

Lotion thermometer. The lotion should be prepared at 38°C (100°F) and injected at body temperature; if it is not the correct temperature the patient is likely to feel giddy and nauseated.

Angular aural forceps.

Wool swabs, and dressed wooden applicators.

Mackintosh.

Towel.
Kidney-shaped receiver.
Receptacles for soiled swabs and instruments.
Head mirror and lamp.

The patient's clothes should be protected by the mackintosh and towel placed round his neck. He should sit upright if possible and hold the kidney dish under the ear.

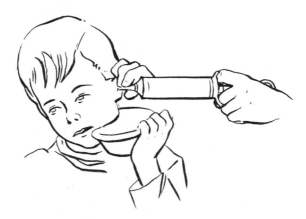

Fig. 25.1. SYRINGING THE EAR, SHOWING METHOD OF HOLDING
THE SYRINGE.

The nurse should wear the head mirror and arrange the lamp so that it will shine on the mirror.

The syringe is filled with the lotion and air expelled.

The pinna of the ear should be pulled upwards and backwards to straighten the meatus and the flow of the lotion directed along the floor of the canal. When a piece of wax has been removed, the ear should be gently cleaned with a piece of wool on the angular forceps and the meatus examined to see if it is clear.

If the wax is hard, drops may be ordered to soften it; sodium bicarbonate or oil may be used.

After syringing a little ointment may be wiped round the meatus to prevent soreness.

A metal ear syringe should be handled with care. If dented, this will interfere with the smooth working of the plunger and there is danger that if force is used in pushing the plunger home, damage to the ear may result. The syringe should always be examined before use, to make sure that the plunger is working smoothly and evenly.

Examination of the Throat and Larynx

Requirements:
Head mirror.
Lamp.
Tongue depressor.
Tongue cloths, folded pieces of gauze, linen or short strips of open wove cotton bandage.
Laryngeal and post-nasal mirrors.
Spirit lamp and matches.
Local anæsthetic.
De Vilbiss spray.
Receptacles for used mirrors and instruments and for soiled swabs.

To Swab or Paint the Throat

Requirements:
Tongue depressor.
Cotton wool swabs on an applicator or held by forceps.
A throat brush may be used in place of wool swabs.
The throat paint and a small gallipot.
Receptacles for used instruments and soiled swabs.
A good light is essential, and a hand lamp or a torch may be required.

The tongue depressor should be placed over the centre of the tongue, pushing it down gently into the floor of the mouth. It should not be placed too far back, as this is likely to make the patient retch.

The applications commonly ordered are glycerin and tannic acid, or Mandl's paint, a preparation of iodine, glycerin and peppermint.

Examination of the Nose and Nasopharynx

Requirements:
Head mirror.
Lamp.

Nasal specula.
Angular dressing forceps.
Post-nasal mirrors.
Tongue depressor.
Spirit lamp and matches.
Cotton wool.
Cotton wool applicators or swab-holding forceps.
Pieces of gauze.
Receptacles for used mirrors and instruments and for soiled
   swabs.

For examinations of the throat, nose and nasopharynx when
the patient is sitting up the nurse should steady the head with a
hand on each side of the forehead, standing behind the patient so
that he does not tend to back away from the examining surgeon.

Probes or wooden applicators dressed with special long-fibre
cotton wool are frequently required in nose and throat work.
These applicators can be bought ready for use or may be prepared
by taking a small flat piece of wool, applying it to the edge of the
applicator and twisting it tightly round, afterwards giving the
wool a pull to make sure that it is firmly applied. Applicators
should be dressed immediately before they are required, if prepared beforehand, they are liable to unwind.

Examination of the Eye

Examination of the interior of the eye with the ophthalmoscope
is a procedure frequently carried out by the doctor in the general
medical wards of a hospital, as well as by the ophthalmic surgeon
in the eye department.

Requirements:
An electrically illuminated ophthalmoscope is usually used.
Small tray with eye drops and dropper.
Small cotton wool swabs or folded lint squares.
Receiver.

The following solutions may be ordered to dilate the pupil
before the examination: homatropine 2 per cent., cocaine 4 per
cent. or a mixture of 2 per cent. homatropine with 1 per cent.
cocaine. No eye drops should be used without specific orders.
The instillation of a mydriatic (a drug which dilates the pupil)
into the eye of a patient suffering from glaucoma may cause

blindness. Eserine drops may be ordered after the examination as a myotic to contract the pupil.

To Instil Drops into the Eye

The patient's head should be tilted well back and he should be directed to look up. One or two drops are then instilled into the lower part of the conjunctival sac, avoiding the cornea, which is the most sensitive part. The patient should be directed to close the

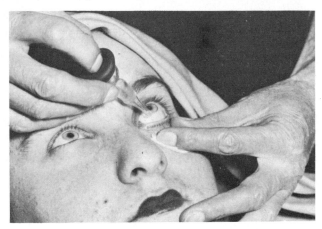

Fig. 25.2. INSTILLATION OF DROPS.

eye for a few minutes. The lids should be gently wiped, taking the swab from the inner to the outer canthus. The dropper should never be allowed to touch the eye or the eyelashes.

To Irrigate the Eye

Requirements:

A special glass irrigator known as an undine.

Lotion at a temperature of 37°C (100°F) 0·9 per cent. sodium chloride, *e.g.* normal saline solution.

Cotton wool or lint swabs.

Mackintosh cape.

Towel.

A receiver for the lotion.

A receptacle for used swabs.

Method. If the patient is in bed, all the pillows but one should be removed so that the patient lies flat with the head tilted back. If he is sitting up in a chair, the head should be tilted back and inclined a little towards the affected side. The towel and mackintosh are arranged to protect the patient's clothing and the receiver arranged to catch the lotion. The patient may hold this himself.

The lotion from the irrigator may be allowed to flow over the

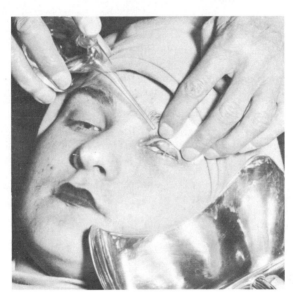

Fig. 25.3. IRRIGATION OF UPPER CONJUNCTIVAL SAC WITH UPPER LID EVERTED.

cheek first, and is then directed in a steady stream from the inner towards the outer canthus of the eye, taking care that the undine does not touch the eye or the eyelashes. It should be held $1\frac{1}{2}$ inches above the eye. The lids should be separated. If they are glued together with sticky discharge, this should be done very gently after well moistening the edges of the lids with lotion. The lids and the surrounding skin should be dried with swabs when the irrigation is completed. An antiseptic ointment for the lids, to be applied after the treatment, may be ordered, such as yellow oxide of mercury. This is applied to the edges of the lids by means of a glass rod.

In all cases where the eye is acutely red or there is any purulent discharge the nurse should observe the following precautions:

(1) She should not directly touch with her fingers either the eye or any articles soiled with the discharge.

(2) If both eyes are to be treated, the cleaner eye should be attended to first.

(3) The nurse's hands must be very thoroughly washed after completing the treatment, the nurse being especially careful not to touch her own eye before doing this.

(4) The patient should be warned not to touch his eyes, and to keep all washing utensils, handkerchiefs and towels separate.

Neurological Examination

The examination of patients suffering from disease or injury of the nervous system includes examination of the interior of the eye by means of an ophthalmoscope and testing of responses to sensory stimuli and reflex muscle responses.

The patient should undress for this examination and wear a pair of short "examination pants".

Requirements:

Patella hammer.

Tuning fork.

Drop bottle containing a mydriatic, such as 2 per cent. homatropine for dilating the pupil of the eye.

Ophthalmoscope.

Tape measure.

Pins.

Cotton wool mops.

Test tube for hot and cold water.

Small bottles containing substances for testing the sense of smell and sense of taste, such as sugar, salt, peppermint.

Skin pencil.

Small soft brush.

Stethoscope.

Sphygmomanometer.

26 RADIOLOGICAL EXAMINATIONS: THE USE OF RADIOACTIVE SUBSTANCES IN DIAGNOSIS AND TREATMENT

Preparation of the Patient for Radiological Examinations

The wishes of the radiologist must be ascertained and carried out in all special examinations, and as several different methods are in use it is only possible to give some indication of the general lines of the preparation in each case.

The patient should be taken to the X-ray department suitably clad, so that the part to be examined can be readily bared of clothing without undue exposure of the patient. If the patient is allowed to keep on one garment during the examination of the chest or abdomen, this garment should be of cotton or flannel and the only fastenings should be tapes. Bone buttons and metal hooks will cast a shadow and linen buttons usually have a metal ring.

Any metal material or substance containing metal salts will obstruct the passage of X-rays and cast a shadow on the film, the only metal which will not materially interfere with the examination is aluminium.

Lead lotion, Elastoplast and kaolin are examples of materials which will obscure the X-ray picture of the underlying tissues. Wet plaster of Paris offers a greater obstruction than the same material when thoroughly dry, so that a plaster splint should, if possible, be allowed to dry before the patient is X-rayed.

It is essential that the patient should remain quite still during the time of the exposure of the film, as any movement renders the radiograph hazy and valueless. The nurse should reassure a nervous patient and endeavour to make him understand that the examination is not in any way painful or harmful.

Examination of the Renal Tract

The aim in the preparation for this examination is to have the intestine emptied of both fæces and flatus, both of which may render the examination useless by obscuring the kidney shadow.

The patient is usually given an aperient such as Dulcolax forty-eight or thirty-six hours before the examination, and kept on a very light diet, or on a strict fluid diet. He is allowed nothing after midnight on the morning of the examination. Charcoal biscuits are sometimes given to absorb the intestinal gas, and an injection of pituitrin may be ordered half an hour before the examination. If the patient is allowed to be out of bed and walking about, there is less likelihood of an accumulation of gas in the intestine than if he is completely confined to bed.

Pyelography

Retrograde Pyelography. A cystoscope is passed into the bladder and a ureteric catheter opaque to X-rays passed along the ureter into the pelvis of the kidney to be examined. The injection of an opaque fluid into the pelvis of the kidney is made through the ureteric catheter. A sterile solution of sodium iodide 10 or 20 per cent. and a water soluble preparation of iodine, iodoxyl (proprietary name, Pyelectan Retrograde) are the two opaque media used for this purpose. The radiographs are taken when the pelvis of the kidney is filled with the solution.

Intravenous Pyelography (Excretion Pyelography). An iodine compound, either diodone or iodoxyl is injected intravenously: when excreted in the urine it is opaque to X-rays, and will therefore cast a shadow of the renal pelves when it fills these structures.

The tray for intravenous injection is taken to the X-ray department with the patient, and the injection made while the patient is on the examination table. Successive films are taken from five minutes after the injection is completed.

Renal Arteriogram. (See pp. 308–309.)

Examination of the Lumbar Spine, Sacrum and Pelvis

The patient is usually prepared as for a renal tract examination.

Examination of the Gall-Bladder

Cholecystography. A radiograph of the gall-bladder may be taken after the same preparation of the patient as that necessary for X-ray of the urinary tract. In addition, however, an examination is carried out after the patient has been given a dye which is excreted in the bile and renders it opaque. This procedure is known as cholecystography. The contrast medium generally used for oral administration is Telepaque, containing 66 per cent. iodine.

The routine followed may vary with the wishes of the radiologist, but the following is an outline of one method used extending over a period of three days.

On the first day a vegetable aperient is given, the dose will depend on the patient's habit with regard to laxatives but should be sufficient to ensure that the bowels act. On the second day the patient takes a low-residue diet excluding green vegetables, cereals and whole-meal bread. After supper the dose of Telepaque is given and no food or drink is allowed until the X-ray film has been taken on the following morning.

The patient attends the X-ray Department at the stated time. He may be required to return after one or two hours for further films. When the gall-bladder, filled with dye containing bile, is demonstrated radiographically, the patient is given a meal with a high fat content, *e.g.* an egg, milk with added cream and a liberal amount of butter on toast or bread. One hour later he attends the department for the final examination.

Intravenous Cholecystogram. When the oral method fails to outline the gall-bladder a cholecystangiography may be performed. This is an examination of the gall-bladder and bile ducts by an intravenous opaque injection (Biligrafin) which contains a higher percentage of iodine than the oral preparation, and results in a higher concentration in the biliary and common bile ducts.

Cholangiography. The bile ducts can be demonstrated by the same intravenous method in patients who have had the gall-bladder removed.

Preparation for Intravenous Cholecystangiography and Cholangiography

1st day. An aperient (vegetable laxative) is given the patient two nights before the X-ray examination.

2nd day. A low residue diet is taken by the patient. No green vegetables, cereals or wholemeal bread. Nothing to eat or drink after midnight.

3rd day. A preliminary film is taken and is examined. If this is satisfactory, *i.e.* if the preparation is adequate and the gall-bladder area is clear of intestinal contents, the intravenous injection is given. The first film is taken 15 minutes later, and films are then taken at varying intervals depending on the rate of concentration of the opaque medium in the gall-bladder. When the concentration is adequate, a fatty meal is given and a further film is taken.

For a cholangiogram films are taken in the same manner up to about 45 minutes after the injection. No fatty meal is given as there is no gall-bladder present.

Examination of the Alimentary Tract

Opaque Meal. The substance used to render the alimentary tract opaque to X-rays is barium sulphate. It is insoluble in water, and therefore is commonly prepared in the form of a suspension containing 4 oz. of barium sulphate in 20 oz. of the preparation.

No aperient should be given within 24 hours of the examination, and any medicine containing bismuth should be discontinued for three days beforehand.

No food or drink should be taken within six hours of the examination. If the examination is for the stomach and duodenum only it may be completed in three hours. If the entire alimentary tract is to be examined, the procedure will extend over 24 or 48 hours, in some cases longer.

As a general rule no food is allowed until the stomach is seen to be empty, and no aperients or other medicines or enemas are allowed until the examination is completed.

An opaque meal examination may be required for an infant, usually in the investigation of pyloric stenosis. In place of the barium preparation 1 oz. of bismuth powder is added to the infant's feed and given at the normal feeding time. No other preparation is required.

Examination of the Appendix

An aperient is given 36 hours before the examination and no food or fluid is allowed within six hours of the barium meal. The first radiograph is taken six hours after the patient has taken the barium mixture and again no food or drink is allowed during this period. Some radiologists order 120 gr. of magnesium sulphate to be given two hours after the barium meal. After the first radiographs the patient may have his normal diet but no aperient may be given until the examination is completed, which is usually at the end of 24 hours.

Opaque Enema

An aperient is given 36 hours before and a colon washout or a Dulcolax suppository four hours before the examination.

The barium mixture for the opaque enema can be conveniently prepared by adding an equal quantity of warm water to the suspension used for the barium meal examination. At least 3 pints will be required.

The enema is allowed to run in slowly through a rectal tube while the radiologist examines the patient under the fluoroscopic screen. The mixture must be at body temperature and should be continually stirred during the administration.

The patient may be required in the X-ray department 24 hours after the enema has been given, and in this case no aperient or enema must be given without special instruction.

The patient is usually allowed a cup of tea on the morning of the examination and his usual diet afterwards.

Bronchography

This examination is carried out after an opaque medium has been injected into the bronchus. The object is to obtain a picture of the bronchi and their branches and is a useful diagnostic aid in suspected carcinoma of the bronchus and in the condition of bronchiectasis. The opaque medium used is an iodine compound

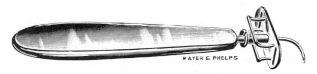

Fig. 26.1. FIELD'S BRONCHOGRAPHY NEEDLE (Child's Size).

in water or in oil; examples of these are Dionosil, Hytrast and Neo-Hydriol. The medium may be introduced in one of three ways:

(1) Through a needle inserted through the cricoid thyroid membrane into the trachea, a method often used for children.

(2) Dropped into the trachea over the back of the tongue, using a syringe and a short curved catheter.

(3) Through a bronchoscope following bronchoscopy.

Preparation of the Patient and Special Precautions

The patient is allowed no food within six hours of the examination if the opaque medium is administered by the oral or intra-tracheal catheter methods on account of the tendency to vomit.

A sedative such as codeine and a hypodermic injection of atropine may be ordered half an hour before the examination.

The patient, with his head supported, should sit on a low chair facing the operator.

After the injection the patient must be warned not to cough until the X-ray films have been taken.

The patient is not allowed any food or fluid until the effects of the local anæsthetic have completely disappeared and the cough reflex is re-established. If the patient tries to swallow while the larynx is still anæsthetized the food or fluid may pass down the trachea into the lungs.

Salpingography

This is an X-ray examination of the Fallopian tube after the injection of iodized oil or diodone viscous solution (Viskiosol Six) into the cavity of the uterus. The object of the examination is to demonstrate the patency of the Fallopian tubes, stenosis or closure of the tubes being one of the causes of sterility in women.

The injection is made on the X-ray table and the patient is usually placed in the lithotomy position. The examination does not as a rule entail any preparation other than the administration of an aperient 36 hours previously if necessary. The patient should empty the bladder immediately before the injection is made.

Radiographs are taken at the completion of the injection and at the end of 24 hours. During this period the patient should not be given an aperient or an enema.

Examinations of the Nervous System

Ventriculography

This examination is carried out after the injection of air into the lateral ventricles of the brain.

The injection of air is carried out by the surgeon in the theatre, and the patient is afterwards transferred to the X-ray department for the radiographs.

The preparation of the patient is the same as for trephining the skull; the scalp must be shaved and the skin prepared.

Encephalography

This is another method of investigating the position and shape of the ventricles. With the patient sitting astride a chair a lumbar puncture is performed. Cerebrospinal fluid is withdrawn and 5 ml. of air is injected. The air rises, as it is lighter than the fluid in the subarachnoid space, and fills the ventricles. The radiographs are then taken.

Myelography

This is an examination of the spinal cord which may be carried out in cases of injury or suspected new growth. An opaque medium, Myodil, is injected through a lumbar or cisternal puncture.

Examination of the Cardiovascular System

Cardiac Catheterization

This procedure is carried out by introducing a long opaque catheter into a vein in the right elbow and watching its passage under the fluorescent screen through the innominate vein, the superior vena cava, the right atrium and the right ventricle to the pulmonary artery. In cases of atrial or ventricular septal defect the catheter may be guided through the hole into the left side of the heart. Blood pressure in the chambers of the heart can be measured and samples of blood are withdrawn for estimation of the oxygen content.

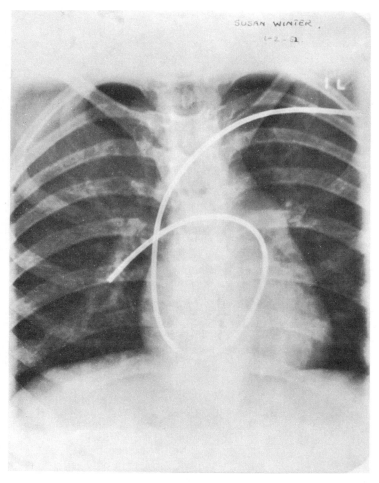

Fig. 26.2. Cardiac Catheterization of the Normal Heart.

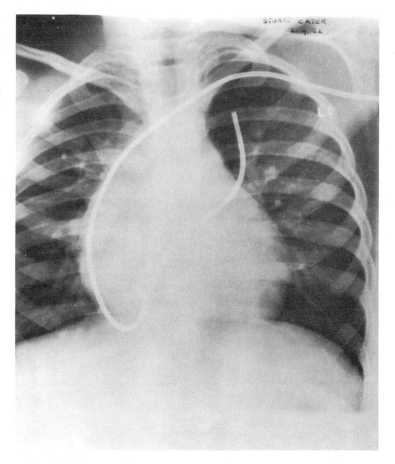

Fig. 26.3. CARDIAC CATHETERIZATION OF HEART WITH ATRIAL SEPTAL
DEFECT.

Angiocardiography

In this examination a radio-opaque dye is injected under pressure into the cardiac catheter. Rapid serial radiograms are taken. Adult patients are usually given a sedative drug before these examinations; a general anæsthetic may be needed for a child.

Arteriography

Arteriography with an opaque medium, Hypaque, is used to demonstrate the blood supply to a particular area; examples of such examinations are:

Femoral Arteriography (Seldinger catheterization)

The introduction of an opaque medium into the arterial circulation via the femoral artery can be used to demonstrate the blood supply to the lower limbs, or, in pregnancy, to the placenta,

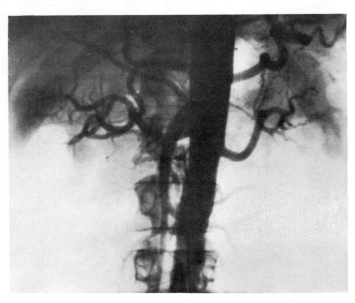

Fig. 26.4. RENAL ARTERIOGRAM.

or to the kidneys (renal arteriography Fig. 26.4). This method may also be used to investigate the left side of the heart.

The patient is prepared for a general anæsthetic. The pubic area is shaved and the skin is cleaned. A Seldinger needle is introduced into the femoral artery and a guide wire is pushed along the artery to the required position. A long catheter is fed over the guide wire, which is then withdrawn, and the opaque medium is injected.

Carotid Arteriography

This examination is used to demonstrate the cerebral blood vessels and is often carried out in cases of subarachnoid hæmorrhage in order to assess the possibility of surgical treatment. The

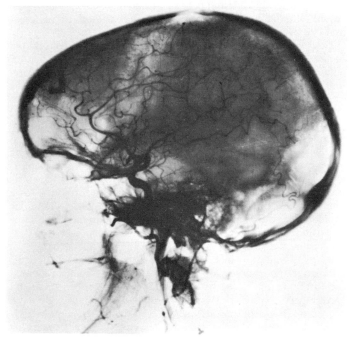

Fig. 26.5. CAROTID ARTERIOGRAM.

opaque medium is introduced into the carotid artery under general anæsthesia.

Therapeutic Use of X-rays

The term "deep X-ray treatment" implies the use of penetrating X-rays produced by the bombardment of a target by electrons travelling at high speed. The source of the energy required for this is high-voltage electricity, of the order of 180,000 to 2 million volts. This form of treatment is most frequently used in cases of malignant growth and many such patients are treated by this method, often in conjunction with surgery.

Many require a large dose spread over a period of several weeks in order that a lethal dose can be delivered at the site of the growth without producing either generalized ill-effects or localized damage to the skin and surrounding tissues.

However carefully the scheme of treatment is devised the tissues surrounding the growth are likely to suffer at least some temporary ill-effects and this is especially true of the skin. Therefore great care is required during and for some weeks after the treatment. The skin of the areas treated must not be subjected to any chemical or physical irritants, therefore washing with soap and water, antiseptic lotions, hot or cold applications and the use of adhesive strappings must be avoided. The skin is less affected by the radiation from "supervoltage" and cobalt units, but in every case the instructions issued by the Radiotherapy Department should be strictly followed. If a male patient is receiving treatment to the face or neck, shaving is usually forbidden for a time and the friction of a closely fitting stiff collar should be avoided. Mucous membrane reacts to radiation in much the same way as skin and some temporary damage to mucus-secreting cells will occur. If the mouth is included in the treatment area there will be a diminution in the secretion of both saliva and mucus. The patient may be very disinclined to eat on account of the discomfort and pain caused by a dry mouth and must be helped and encouraged as much as possible. Frequent non-irritating fluids to drink and frequent mouth washes will help. If the mouth is painful, lozenges containing a local anæsthetic—e.g. benzocaine —may be ordered, or aspirin gargles may give relief.

If an ulcerating malignant growth is being treated, the discharge is likely to be both offensive and profuse, and therefore frequent changes of dressings are necessary.

The patient's blood count is taken daily or at frequent intervals. A falling white cell count may be treated by drugs which increase the production of white cells, *e.g.* Prednisolone. In some cases radiation treatment may be suspended.

General effects of radiation are not usually marked when divided dosage is used spread over a period of weeks, but were fairly common in the early days of X-ray treatment when a single large dose was used. However, some patients may complain of loss of appetite, nausea, inability to sleep and general depression.

Radium Therapy

Radium is a naturally occurring element which spontaneously emits radiations of short wave-length. Radium is chiefly used in the form of its salt, radium sulphate, and in the form of the emanation or gas (radon) which is given off from it. The salt is placed in needles or sometimes in larger containers and the emanation is collected in radon "seeds".

Methods of Application

Surface Application. The needles or applicators are embedded in a suitable mould made of Columba paste or Stent's dental composition, or may be attached to sorbo rubber or other suitable material which can be accurately applied to the desired area.

Interstitial Irradiation. Needles or radon seeds are inserted into the tissues.

Cavitary Irradiation. Applicators are placed inside natural cavities of the body—*e.g.* the vagina, cervical canal and the body of the uterus.

Rules and Precautions to be Observed in the Handling of Radium

Radium needles or containers, including radon seeds, should never be touched by hand but must always be manipulated with long-handled forceps the handles of which are covered with rubber. When radium is removed from the safe and carried to and from the theatre a lead-lined box with a long carrying handle should be used for its transport.

The threading of needles and the preparation of applicators

must be carried out on a special table provided with a lead screen. Proximity to the radium must be for as short a time as possible.

The time at which the radium treatment is begun and the time at which it is due to be terminated must be carefully noted. The success of the treatment and the safety of the patient depend on careful calculation of the dosage to be employed. The time during which the radium is in contact with the tissues is one factor in these calculations.

Careful checking of the radium is essential. The amount of radium, the number and size of the needles used are entered on a record card; unused containers are checked and returned to the radium safe.

Radioactive Isotopes

Isotopes are variations of an element which have identical chemical properties but different atomic weights. Most elements have at least two isotopes. The radioactive isotopes of certain elements which are now being used in medical treatment are artificially produced by the bombardment of the nuclei of the atoms in an atomic pile. The radioactive isotopes used in medicine are in fact by-products of the atomic research stations.

Examples of the medical use of radioactive isotopes:

Radioactive iodine in the treatment of carcinoma of the thyroid gland and thyrotoxicosis. In the latter condition most authorities consider that radioactive iodine should not be given to patients under 40 years of age. The radioactive iodine is given by mouth and absorbed into the blood stream from the alimentary tract. From the blood it is deposited in the thyroid gland and there acts as a source of localized radiation.

Radioactive phosphorus. This substance has been found to be effective in the treatment of polycythæmia, a condition in which the blood contains an excessive number of red cells. The phosphorus may be given by mouth or by intravenous injection.

Radioactive cobalt. This has a long "life" compared with most other radioactive isotopes. It is now being used in place of radium or as an alternative to deep X-ray in a "bomb" or beam unit in the treatment of malignant disease.

Radioactive gold. This isotope is used locally in the peritoneal or pleural cavities in cases of malignant disease where secondary deposits cause large peritoneal or pleural effusions necessitating frequent aspiration.

Radioactive Tracers

Radioactive isotopes are useful assistants in solving physiological and medical problems. Very minute quantities can be traced in the body by means of a delicate instrument, the Geiger counter. For example, radioactive iodine is used to assess the activity of the thyroid gland. A small dose is given by mouth and the Geiger counter is set up in position over the thyroid area and will record the arrival of the radioactive isotope in the tissues of the gland. If there is no active thyroid tissue no iodine will be taken up; if there is enlargement and/or increased activity of the gland the absorption of the iodine will be more rapid than normal.

Precautions

All persons working with radioactive substances or X-rays must observe the regulations laid down for their protection or their health will sooner or later be affected. Prolonged exposure to even small doses of radiation will damage the bone marrow and eventually diminish the supply of blood cells. The germ plasm of the ovaries and testes is damaged by radiation and sterility may result. In the early days of the use of X-rays repeated exposure of the hands caused destruction of the skin, ulceration and later malignant changes.

In the handling of radioactive isotopes similar precautions are required as in dealing with other forms of radiation, but in addition there is the danger of contamination with radioactive particles.

When patients are receiving doses of radioactive iodine some of the material will be excreted in the urine. Nursing staff dealing with bed-pans and urinals should wear protective clothing and rubber gloves. Should there be any suspicion of contamination of the hands or any skin area a thorough washing with soap and water must be immediately carried out. The radioactive urine must not be emptied directly into the sewerage system. The radioactivity, however, rapidly decays (the exact period of time which must elapse before the isotope is inactive varies with the different elements), and after storage for the appropriate length of time the urine can be discarded. Urine awaiting disposal can be stored in suitable large bottles or tanks in lead-lined cupboards.

The following regulations are an example of the precautions which the nursing staff must observe in caring for a patient who is receiving treatment of the thyroid gland with radioactive iodine.

China. Separate china and cutlery will be used for all patients having had radioactive iodine. The china is green-bordered. All cutlery and glassware is marked with green paint. It may be washed in the kitchen, but in different water from other china. A separate dish mop and towel will be used and all cutlery is to be soaked in half strength 1 per cent. potassium iodide for $\frac{1}{4}$ hour before being washed.

Mouthwash utensils. All utensils are marked with green paint.

Urine. Each patient has his own marked bed-pan. Urine is placed by patients in, and saved in, 24 hourly bottles behind lead shielding until it is safe for disposal. These urine bottles are then dealt with by the laboratory staff.

Fæces. No precautions are required.

Vomit and sputum. Any material vomited or expectorated within the first 48 hours of a dose is saved in a lead-lined cupboard, until the radioactive isotope has decayed to a safe level.

Contaminated bedding, etc. This is saved for monitoring, any urine spills being notified.

Hands. In order to avoid contamination of the hands rubber gloves are worn when attending to patients who are receiving therapy doses. The gloves must be worn for bed-making and for giving attention to the patient during the first 3 days after a therapeutic dose and during the first 7 days when dealing with the patient's urine. Gloves should be washed on the hands before they are removed. The hands must be washed after removing the gloves and again before eating or smoking.

Nurses should avoid exposing their hands for longer than a minute or two to the radiation from the neck region.

27 PREPARATION FOR SPECIAL EXAMINATIONS AND PROCEDURES

This chapter describes the preparation of the apparatus and the care of the patient in relation to some special investigations and procedures which are commonly carried out in the ward by the doctor. It can be assumed that most, if not all, of the items listed below will normally be needed and therefore in describing each individual procedure *only the special instruments or apparatus required will be mentioned.*

General Requirements

   (1) Skin cleansing agent, *e.g.* 1 per cent. cetrimide.
   (2) 1 or 2 ml. syringe and needles for local anæsthetic.
   (3) Local anæsthetic, *e.g.* 0·5 per cent. lignocaine.
   (4) Instrument handling forceps.
   (5) Sterile towels, swabs and dressings.
   (6) Sterile rubber gloves of suitable size.
   (7) Sterile dressing, forceps and scissors.
   (8) Sterile scalpel, or small knife blade and handle.
   (9) Sterile containers for laboratory specimens.
  (10) Pathological examination request forms and labels.
  (11) Mackintoshes or protective sheeting.
  (12) Collodion, adhesive strapping and scissors.
  (13) Receptacles for used instruments and dressings.

Exploration and Aspiration of the Chest for Fluid in the Pleural Cavity

Exploration and, where necessary, aspiration of the pleural cavity are used in diagnosis and the treatment of a pleural effusion. Such an effusion may be an inflammatory exudate as in pleurisy accompanying pneumonia, or a transudate such as the fluid which collects as part of a generalized œdema in congestive heart failure.

Requirements:
General requirements as listed above.
10 or 20 ml. exploring syringe and long needles.
Two-way tap to fit the syringe.
Tubing to fit the tap.
2 sterile measure jugs.

Martin's syringe is one type of two-way syringe used for aspiration of the chest. This syringe has a bayonet fitting and is supplied with a trocar and cannula and a sharp needle. A piece of rubber tubing is attached to one arm of the nozzle through which the fluid drawn up into the syringe is ejected into the measure jug.

Preparation of the Patient

The patient should sit well forward in the bed with his head flexed and his arms resting on a pillow placed on a bedtable in front of him. The pillows behind him must be removed so that the doctor has easy access to the patient's back. The skin over the area where the puncture will be made is cleaned and the local anæsthetic injected.

Pleural Biopsy

Biopsy of the parietal pleura is most commonly undertaken in order to determine whether a pleural effusion is of tuberculous or malignant origin.

Requirements:
General requirements as listed on page 315.
Abram's pleural biopsy needle (Fig. 27.1).
Aspirating syringe.
Two-way tap to fit the syringe.
Skin suture.

Preparation of the Patient

The biopsy needle is usually inserted into the posterior chest wall, the actual site of the puncture being determined by physical and radiological examination. The patient should sit forward in the bed in the position described under "pleural aspiration". No preparation other than cleaning the skin and the injection of a local anæsthetic is usually required and there are usually no after effects, although the patient may experience some aching pain in the chest.

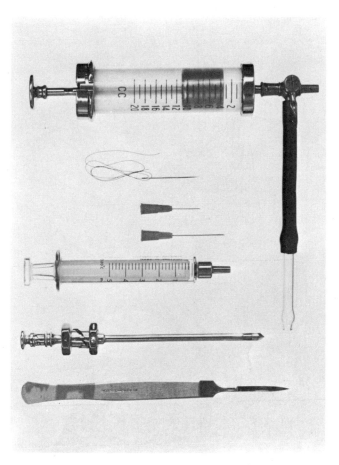

Fig. 27.1. PLEURAL BIOPSY SET.

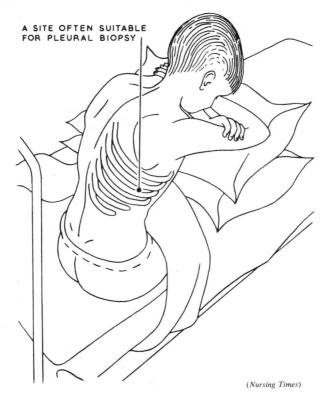

A SITE OFTEN SUITABLE
FOR PLEURAL BIOPSY

(*Nursing Times*)

Fig. 27.2. POSITION OF THE PATIENT FOR PLEURAL BIOPSY.

The small skin incision is closed with a single suture and a small sterile dressing is applied.

Tapping the Peritoneal Cavity (Paracentesis Abdominis)

Tapping may be needed in order to withdraw fluid from the peritoneal cavity (ascites) in cases of cardiac or liver diseases and in malignant conditions.

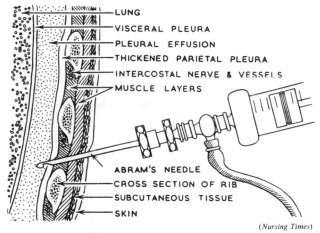

LUNG
VISCERAL PLEURA
PLEURAL EFFUSION
THICKENED PARIETAL PLEURA
INTERCOSTAL NERVE & VESSELS
MUSCLE LAYERS
ABRAM'S NEEDLE
CROSS SECTION OF RIB
SUBCUTANEOUS TISSUE
SKIN

(*Nursing Times*)

Fig. 27.3. THE CHEST WALL AND PENETRATION OF THE PLEURAL BIOPSY NEEDLE.

Requirements:
General requirements as listed on page 315.
Ascites trocar and cannula (Fig. 27.4).

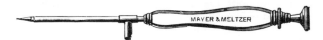

MAYER & MELTZER

Fig. 27.4. THOMPSON'S ASCITES TROCAR AND CANNULA.

Tubing to fit side outlet,
or Southey's trocar and cannula with fine rubber tubing
(Fig. 27.5).
Many-tailed bandage or abdominal binder.
Pail or other receptacle to stand at the side of the bed for the
fluid.
When the Southey's tube is used the trocar should have the
small shield screwed into place and the tubing should be attached
to the end of the cannula. The trocar should be pushed through
the rubber tubing (holding this stretched) so that its end protrudes
just below the end of the cannula.

It is important that the fine tubing should be new and in good condition; if at all perished it will lose its elasticity, and therefore the small hole made by the trocar will not close up when the trocar is removed.

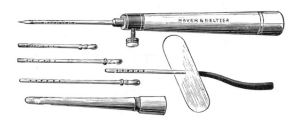

Fig. 27.5. SOUTHEY'S TROCAR AND CANNULAE.

Preparation of the Patient

Immediately before the tapping the bladder must be emptied and catheterization may be needed.

The patient should sit upright supported with pillows. The bandage or binder should be placed in position so that it can be applied as soon as the trocar and cannula are inserted. If a large trocar and cannula are used, the fluid drains quickly and the nurse should tighten the binder frequently. If a Southey's tube is used the fluid drains much more slowly. Two small pieces of adhesive strapping will be required to keep the small shield in position.

Tapping the Legs

The commoner causes of gross œdema of the legs are cardiac failure and nephritis.

Requirements:

General requirements as listed on page 315.

Southey's small trocars and cannulæ (two for each leg are usually required).

Fine rubber drainage tubing.

Suitable containers, *e.g.* bottles or jars, into which the fluid drains.

The tubing is fitted on to the cannulæ as for paracentesis

abdominis with Southey's tubes, but the small metal shields are omitted.

Preparation of the Patient

As a general rule an endeavour is made to drain fluid from other parts of the body into the legs prior to the tapping. To achieve this the patient's legs should hang down below the level of the trunk for two or three days beforehand.

The skin on the outer aspect of the legs is prepared.

A local anæsthetic may be injected into the skin surrounding the site for the insertion of the cannulæ.

When the tubes have been inserted, small pieces of gauze are slipped under the ends of the cannulæ to prevent pressure on the skin. The tubes are kept in place by small pieces of adhesive strapping and covered by sterile dressings. The ends of the rubber drainage tubes are placed in the jars.

The tubes may be left in for twenty-four hours or longer; during this time the dressings should be changed twice a day, or more often if necessary. After the tubes have been removed the punctures must be covered with sterile dressings until they are healed.

As an alternative method, small scarifications may be made in the œdematous tissue and the fluid then drains into large dressings.

Lumbar Puncture

Lumbar puncture is carried out in order to obtain samples of cerebrospinal fluid and to measure the pressure of the fluid. The procedure is also used when drugs are given by intrathecal injection.

Requirements:

General requirements as listed on page 315.

Lumbar puncture needles. If the pressure of the cerebrospinal fluid is to be measured, a needle with a tap and side piece is used. A small piece of rubber tubing to fit the side piece and the glass manometer will be required.

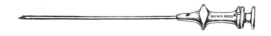

Fig. 27.6. Barker's Needle for Lumbar Puncture.

If drugs are to be injected a large record syringe and an adaptor to fit the lumbar puncture needle will be required.

A general anæsthetic may be required if the patient is restless or likely to have fits.

Position of the Patient

Usually the procedure is carried out with the patient lying on his side near the edge of the bed. The spine and the legs are flexed as far as possible in order to separate the intervertebral spaces. The usual site for the puncture is between the third and fourth lumbar vertebræ. In some cases the patient may be sitting up with the knees and spine flexed.

After the procedure the patient should be kept quiet and lying flat for several hours, as severe headache is likely to occur. This may be treated by raising the foot of the bed.

When specimens of the cerebrospinal fluid are required for pathological examination, these should be taken to the laboratory immediately.

Cisternal Puncture

The requirements are the same as for lumbar puncture, except that a special needle with the shaft marked in centimetres may be used.

The site for this puncture is the junction of the skull with the spine, and the skin over the area will usually require shaving.

Venesection

While venesection is most commonly performed to obtain blood for transfusion, this procedure may also be used in the treatment of certain disorders in order to reduce the blood volume. Examples of such conditions are polycythæmia, a condition in which both the number of red cells and the total volume of the blood are increased, and in cardiac disease with pulmonary œdema, where the withdrawal of 300 ml. or more of blood relieves the congestion in the right side of the heart.

Requirements:

General requirements as listed on page 315.

Venesection needle, adaptor and tubing. The standard blood donor "taking set" is often used.

Sphygmomanometer.

Bandages.

Preparation of the Patient

The usual site for venesection is one of the superficial veins on the anterior surface of the elbow. The sphygmomanometer cuff is applied to the arm, as high above the elbow as possible, and inflated until the manometer reads between 60 and 80 mm. and the superficial veins are distended. The doctor then inserts the venesection needle and blood flows into the bottle. The patient is asked to open and close his fist in order to assist the flow of blood. If the blood is being collected for transfusion, the bottle will contain an anticoagulant solution and an assistant should shake the bottle gently while the blood flows, so that it mixes with the solution. A specimen of blood for testing is collected in the sample bottle provided.

Where venesection is required in the treatment of disease this blood is not used subsequently for transfusion purposes.

When the needle is withdrawn a small dressing is applied to the puncture and secured with a firm bandage to prevent the formation of a hæmatoma.

Collection of blood from donors for transfusion is usually undertaken by the Blood Transfusion Services. Donors should lie flat for about 15 minutes after they have given blood and be given about ½ pint of fluid to drink; tea or coffee are usually the most acceptable drinks. At the end of a further fifteen minutes the donor is usually allowed to leave.

Bone Marrow Biopsy

In the investigation of some diseases of the blood a specimen of the red bone marrow is required and this is obtained either from the sternum or the iliac crest.

Requirements:

General requirements as listed on page 315.

2 ml. aspirating syringe.

Sternal puncture needle with stilette. This is a hollow needle with a short bevelled point and an adjustable "stop" or guard (Fig. 27.7).

The patient is usually given a sedative, *e.g.* Seconal 200 mg. or Physeptone 10 mg. three-quarters to one hour before the procedure is carried out.

The patient should lie flat with the head extended and a small pillow under the shoulders.

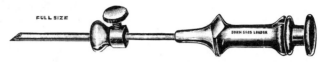

Fig. 27.7. STERNAL PUNCTURE NEEDLE.

Splenic Aspiration

Splenic aspiration is sometimes performed in cases of un-explained splenomegaly and in some blood diseases. For this a fine-gauge Harris's lumbar puncture needle may be used, and a syringe for aspirating the specimen.

Liver Biopsy

Biopsy may be required in the investigation of liver disorders where physical and laboratory examinations have failed to give a diagnosis.

Requirements:

General requirements as listed on page 315.

Liver biopsy needle, *e.g.* Silverman's or a modification of this type (see Fig. 27.8), or Menghini's needle (Fig. 27.9).

Fine injection needle, 3 inches in length.

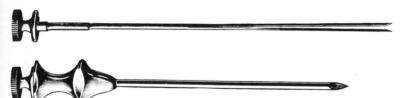

Fig. 27.8. SILVERMAN'S LIVER BIOPSY NEEDLE, ADULT SIZE.

Preparation of the Patient

The patient's blood group is ascertained and his blood is cross-matched. The hæmoglobin content, bleeding and clotting times and the prothrombin content of the blood are estimated. The examination is not usually carried out if the prothrombin content is below 70 per cent. of the normal.

Procedure

The patient lies on his back well over to the right side of the bed, the trunk is then slightly tilted to the right by placing a pillow under his left side.

Following the biopsy it is important to keep a close watch on the patient's condition as hæmorrhage may occur. A pulse chart should be kept for at least twelve hours.

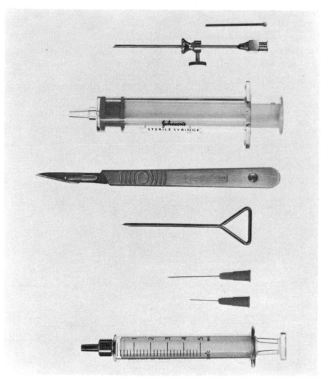

Fig. 27.9. MENGHINI'S LIVER BIOPSY SET.

Renal Biopsy

Renal biopsy may be useful in elucidating some cases of renal disease when other methods have failed to give a definite diagnosis.

The biopsy specimen is obtained by using a modified type of the Silverman's liver biopsy needle.

Preparation of the Patient

An X-ray examination is carried out in order to determine the size and position of the kidneys. The patient's blood group is identified and his blood is cross-matched in case a transfusion is needed. The hæmoglobin is also estimated.

The site of the biopsy is usually the lower pole of the right kidney. The patient lies in the prone position with a sandbag under the abdomen, this fixes the kidney against the dorsal surface of the body and helps to reduce the risk of hæmorrhage.

The position of the kidney is determined after the injection of a local anæsthetic, by a fine exploring needle.

After renal biopsy has been performed it is important to keep a close watch for bleeding; a certain amount of hæmaturia is common, but even if slight it should be reported immediately.

USES AND APPLICATION OF HEAT, COLD AND MEDICATED PREPARATIONS

Heat applied externally dilates the surface blood vessels and increases the blood supply to the superficial tissues, encouraging the removal of inflammatory exudate and reducing swelling. Heat also produces relaxation of the muscles. It is therefore a simple and useful method of relieving pain and congestion. A hot water bottle, or a hot bath, can be very comforting and often effective in relieving stiff and aching joints and muscles. Where deep penetration of heat is ordered in the treatment of arthritic joints, or to hasten the resolution of inflammation, it is usually prescribed in the form of "short wave" diathermy which is given by the physiotherapist. Steam inhalations are a useful form of local treatment for sinusitis, tracheitis and other respiratory tract infections.

Cold depletes the local circulation and increases muscle tone. Cold applications, therefore, may be used to prevent swelling, for example, in the treatment of such injuries as sprains and strains of the soft tissues around a joint. Cold will also relieve some types of pain, an example of this being the use of an icebag to relieve headache.

Hot Applications

Hot Water Bottles

A rubber hot water bottle used as a local application of heat must be well protected with a thick cover which should enclose the stopper. It should be filled with water hot enough to be felt as comfortable warmth when the bottle is covered, not higher than 82°C (180°F) and never with boiling water. The bottle should always be tested for leakage after filling and before it is given to the patient. It should be remembered that a patient suffering acute pain, for example gall-stone colic, will not notice a lesser discomfort and therefore great care must be taken to guard against burns in such cases.

Some hospitals prohibit the use of hot water bottles for any purpose and everyone agrees that they should not be given to young children or to restless, confused or unconscious patients, or to those who have loss of sensation or of the power of movement. The hot water bottle is, however, a simple form of treatment likely to be available in the home and if used with proper care should not be a danger in the majority of instances where the application of heat can give relief.

Kaolin Poultice (Cataplasma Kaolini)

The basis of this application is china clay, which contains, in addition, glycerin, menthol and methyl salicylate. It has analgesic as well as heat-retaining properties.

The kaolin poultice may be left on six to twelve hours, and this is a great advantage in cases where frequent applications are exhausting to the patient, and it has also the advantage of being light in weight.

Requirements:

Tin containing cataplasma kaolini.
Saucepan containing boiling water.
Lint or old linen.
Palette knife.
Jug containing boiling water.
Poultice board.
Warmed plates, trays or dishes to carry the poultice to the bedside.

Place the tin containing the application in the saucepan and allow it to heat by keeping the water simmering for about twenty minutes. The contents of the tin should be stirred occasionally, so that the material is evenly heated all through.

Spread the poultice smoothly on the lint or linen, place it on a warm tray or plate, covered (do not roll or fold the poultice), and take it to the bedside. The heat of the application should be tested on the back of the hand before applying. Clay holds the heat for a long time, and unless the poultice is tested to make sure that it is not too hot there is a danger of burning the patient.

Fomentation

A fomentation is a simple method of applying heat locally but does not retain the heat for any length of time.

Requirements:

A piece of flannel of double or treble thickness.

A piece of protective material, such as jaconet or polythene sheeting, $\frac{1}{2}$ inch larger all round than the flannel.

A piece of Gamgee or cotton wool $\frac{1}{2}$ inch larger than the jaconet.

A wringer made of strong cotton or linen material. In the home a strong kitchen towel makes a good wringer.

A bowl.

A kettle of boiling water.

A flannel bandage or binder should be used to keep the application in position.

Place the flannel in the centre of the wringer and take care that the ends of the wringer lie outside the bowl, pour the boiling water over the flannel and wringer and then wring the flannel as dry as possible. Give it a quick shake to allow the steam to escape before applying.

The flannel is then covered with the jaconet and wool and bandaged in position.

The frequency with which the fomentation is changed will depend upon its size and thickness and the condition for which it is ordered. In some cases it will require changing every half-hour, in others every two hours will be sufficient.

When a fomentation is to be changed, the fresh application should be prepared and the old one removed (leaving the part covered with the piece of wool) before wringing out the fresh fomentation.

Steam Inhalations

Steam Kettle

The kettle may be used in conjunction with a tent bed in the treatment of bronchitis. In a small room a screen round the head of the bed with a sheet over the top may replace the full tent. An electric kettle is used, if available, as there is a risk of fire if a spirit stove is used for heating.

The kettle should stand on a stool and the spout should be introduced either at the side or the back of the tent.

The kettle should be filled with boiling water, and if a drug is ordered this is added to the water in the prescribed quantity. Compound tincture of benzoin is commonly used. The kettle usually requires filling every two hours, and should be refilled with boiling water. The air temperature in the tent should be 21°C (70°F).

If the patient is a child it is necessary to have some form of restraint, so that the child cannot get at any part of the kettle or come into close contact with the steam, or else the kettle should be sufficiently far from the cot to prevent this occurring.

Nelson's Inhaler

The earthenware inhaler should be half filled with boiling water to which the prescribed amount of menthol or tincture of benzoin is added. This is usually 60 minims of tincture of benzoin or a few crystals of menthol to 1 pint of water.

A flannel cover should be placed round the inhaler and the patient's shoulders should be covered with a shawl or small blanket. The patient is directed to put his lips to the mouth-piece and breathe in through the mouth and out through the nose.

A very satisfactory inhaler can be made by using a quart jug with a small towel twisted round the rim. The patient is directed to rest his mouth on the towel and breathe in the steam.

Some authorities recommend that the hot water in the inhaler should not be hotter than 82°C (180°F). A steam inhalation is not suitable for a patient who for any reason is unable to co-operate in the treatment.

Cold Applications

Cold Compress

Requirements:

A double piece of lint or old linen cut to the required size.

Ice-cold water or lead lotion.

An open-wove gauze bandage.

If the patient is in bed, a piece of protective sheeting should be placed under the limb and a bed cradle will be required over the limb.

The compress is wrung out of the lotion, applied to the part and secured with the gauze bandage. Both compress and bandage must be kept moistened with the water or lotion.

Ice Bag

Requirements:

Chipped ice.

Ice pick.

Salt.

Ice bag.

A flannel cover for the bag or a piece of lint.

A bed cradle.

The bag is one-third filled with chipped ice to which 1 or 2 teaspoonfuls of salt have been added. The air is expelled and the bag carefully dried outside.

It is then placed in the flannel cover and suspended so that it rests lightly on the skin. It may be convenient to suspend the bag from a cradle.

It must be refilled as soon as the ice has melted.

If an ice bag is not obtainable, a rubber sponge bag or a polythene bag can be used as a substitute, but care must be taken to suspend it in such a manner that it cannot spill the contents.

Medicated Preparations

A large number of medicated preparations in the form of lotions, pastes, creams, paints, emulsions and ointments are used in the treatment of skin conditions.

Ointments (*e.g.* Whitfield's (benzoic acid compound) Dithranol and hydrocortisone ointments). Some ointments, such as Whitfield's, need to be rubbed into the skin; others are spread on strips of soft material, such as old linen or cotton sheeting.

Paints and emulsions (*e.g.* gentian violet paint used in the treatment of pyogenic skin infection and benzyl benzoate emulsion used in the treatment of scabies). Paints and emulsions are applied directly on to the skin using a brush or a wool swab.

Before benzyl benzoate emulsion is applied the patient is given a hot bath to soften the skin and open the burrows of the parasite. The emulsion is then applied to the skin from the neck to the toes, using a wide brush. Twenty-four hours later a second application is given. On the evening of the following day the patient has a hot bath and puts on clean clothing.

Creams and pastes (*e.g.* calamine and coal tar pastes or creams) may be spread on strips of soft material or applied directly to the skin using the finger tips or a wooden spatula.

Lotions (*e.g.* lead, calamine, hydrocortisone lotions) can be applied as wet dressings; strips of old linen or cotton sheeting are soaked in the lotion and squeezed to remove excess moisture. The dressings should be kept moist.

Keeping extensive dressings in position is often a problem. Tubular gauze is useful for the limbs and trunk and this type of bandage can also be used for the face as a mask, or for the scalp as a cap. If roller bandages are used they should be light in weight, *e.g.* open-wove cotton gauze and should be firmly applied. Loose bandages may rub the skin and as they entangle air, they will be hot and irritating.

Starch Poultice

A starch poultice may be used to soften and aid the removal of crusts and scabs in some skin conditions, *e.g.* impetigo.

Requirements:

A sufficient quantity of powdered starch.

Boric powder.

Old linen cut to the required size.

Boiling water.

Cold water.

A board.

A mixing bowl.

A spoon.

A palette knife.

A small saucepan.

Jaconet or any protective material.

Bandages. If applied to the head, a cotton cap or a triangular bandage is convenient.

Measure the starch into the mixing bowl ($1\frac{1}{2}$ tablespoonfuls for every $\frac{1}{2}$ pint of water used will give the required consistency when cooked) and mix with it 1 teaspoonful of boric powder.

Break up the starch with sufficient cold water to make a thick paste, add the boiling water, and stir well until the starch turns clear. Pour the mixture into the saucepan and boil for two minutes.

Allow to cool slightly and then spread it evenly on the linen about $\frac{3}{4}$ inch thick.

When applied, the poultice should be almost cold and have the consistency of a jelly.

Cover with the protective material and bandage into position. The application is left on for six to twelve hours.

When the poultice is taken off the scabs should be gently removed with dressing forceps and warm olive oil.

Medicated Preparations Used as Supporting Dressings for Varicose Ulcers

Varicose ulcers, as the name suggests, occur in patients with varicosity of the superficial veins of the leg, particularly if they have suffered attacks of thrombo-phlebitis. The ulcers commonly begin just above the medial malleolus, but may spread right round the leg. These ulcers are painful, disabling and often slow to heal. The usual treatment is to apply a supporting dressing and a firm bandage from the base of the toes to just below the knee; examples of two methods used are:

Viscopaste bandages. These bandages are impregnated with gelatin and zinc oxide powder, they are supplied ready for use. Padding is needed over the Achilles tendon behind the heel and over the malleoli; a gauze dressing is applied over the ulcerated area. The bandage begins with a circular turn round the foot and then when the foot and heel are covered, the bandage is taken up the leg. No pleats or reverse turns should be made; where necessary the edge of the bandage is cut to fit the contours of the leg.

Bisgard's Treatment. Bisgard's solution containing 1 per cent. aluminium acetate and 3 per cent. boric acid is applied as a wet dressing using twenty layers of gauze in order to ensure that the dressing is really wet. It is covered with a protective layer of oiled silk or non-absorbent wool. Wool padding is required behind the Achilles tendon of the heel and the lateral and medial malleoli. The leg is then firmly bandaged from the toes to the knee with an elastic webbing bandage. The patient is shown how to carry out the treatment at home. Each evening she removes the old dressing, massages the whole leg and the area around the ulcer before applying a fresh dressing which can be kept in place at night by a gauze bandage. In the morning a fresh dressing is applied and covered with the elastic webbing bandage which must be worn all day.

The patient is instructed to walk as much as possible but to avoid standing.

29 METHODS OF TREATMENT BY BATHS AND SPONGING

Most of us regard a bath as an efficient and pleasant way of keeping our skin clean, and because of the relaxing and sedative effect of a warm bath we often choose to take it just before bedtime. For these reasons the patient too, whether in hospital or in his own home, usually appreciates a daily warm bath as soon as his condition permits.

Baths may also be ordered as a form of treatment, for example in some skin conditions, or as a means of warming or cooling a patient.

Hot Baths

A hot bath given for its cleansing and sedative effect is usually prepared at a temperature of 40° to 43°C (104° to 110°F). The temperature will depend to some extent on the individual; some people like to steam and soak in really hot water, but in the case of elderly or feeble patients a temperature of 40°C should not as a rule be exceeded. A warm bath at a temperature of 35° to 38°C (95° to 100°F) may be ordered to resuscitate a new-born infant with a low body temperature, or in the treatment of infantile convulsions for its soothing effect.

A really hot bath produces muscular relaxation, dilates the superficial blood vessels and interferes with heat loss. It is therefore often useful in relieving pain and stiffness following strenuous physical exertion, but can cause faintness and collapse. In a patient enfeebled by illness there is even a risk of him becoming unconscious and drowning in the bath. An elderly patient, or one who is only just convalescent, should not be left alone in the bathroom. If a patient is considered fit enough to bath himself, the bathroom door should be left unlocked and after two or three minutes the nurse should make sure that he is not in need of help.

The duration of the bath will depend on the individual and on the reason for the bath; it may be from three to fifteen minutes.

Cold Baths

A cold bath at room temperature about 18°C (65°F) increases muscle tone and cools the surface of the body. Vigorous drying with a rough towel after a cold bath produces a warm glowing feeling, but generally cold baths are suitable only for healthy individuals.

Reduction of Body Temperature

Immersion in cold or iced water can be used to reduce the body temperature. This treatment is now seldom used to reduce the temperature of a febrile patient; sponging, which will be described later, is more suitable for this purpose. The iced water bath is, however, used to reduce a normal body temperature to subnormal levels (hypothermia) in order to slow metabolism and reduce the oxygen needs of the cells. Hypothermia may be used in the treatment of patients with severe head injuries or, in conjunction with anæsthesia, in cardiac and brain surgery. In the latter case an immersion bath is not a very convenient method and other means of reducing the temperature can be used, for example the "heat exchange" apparatus, which may be combined with extracorporeal oxygenation of the blood in open heart operations. Here the blood is withdrawn from the body and after oxygenation it is passed through tubes which are surrounded by a jacket containing cold water before it is returned to the circulation. In moderate hypothermia the body temperature is reduced to 28° to 30°C (82° to 86°F).

The nurse will realize that hypothermia is a specialized form of treatment and calls for very careful control, whatever method of cooling is used. Where the iced water bath is used for this purpose the doctor will give precise instructions and will supervise the procedure.

Medicated Baths

Medicated baths are not now often used but may be ordered in generalized skin conditions with the object of cleansing the skin and allaying irritation. Baths used in the treatment of skin lesions are usually given tepid (about 29°C (85°F)). The duration of the bath may be 10 to 15 minutes, or longer.

Sterile Saline Baths. Sterile 0·9 per cent. sodium chloride baths are sometimes used in the treatment of burns to clean the area or to soak off adherent dressings.

Alkaline Baths. 4 ounces of sodium bicarbonate ($\frac{1}{2}$ cupful) is added to a tepid bath. This bath may be ordered to alleviate itching, for instance in pruritus. In pruritus of the vulva or the anal region a sitz bath, or hip bath, may be used.

Starch Bath. One ounce of powdered starch is required for each gallon of water used. The starch powder is mixed to paste with cold water, then sufficient boiling water is poured on the paste to make a mucilage which is added to the tepid water in the bath. A starch bath is a soothing treatment which may be used in the treatment of generalized eczema.

Sponging

This form of treatment may be ordered for febrile patients if the temperature rises to 40°C (104°F) or over, or if the patient feels hot, uncomfortable and restless although his temperature is only moderately high. To be effective, sponging must be carried out with the least possible exertion on the part of the patient. The object of the treatment is to increase heat loss by evaporation and a successful sponge will reduce the temperature about one degree Centigrade (two degrees Fahrenheit). It is not a drastic form of treatment and, if carried out skilfully, can have no ill-effects.

Requirements:

A large washing bowl.

Jugs of hot and cold water.

A bath thermometer.

At least two sponges, or pieces of soft towelling. If the temperature is very high the treatment will be more effective if additional sponges are used, one in the nape of the neck, one in each axilla, under each hand and under each knee joint. These sponges are changed as they become warm.

A towel.

A long mackintosh or piece of protective sheeting.

Two cotton blankets or large bath towels.

The top bedclothes are removed, the protective sheeting and one cotton blanket, or towel, are rolled under the patient. The nightgown is removed and the patient is covered with the second blanket.

The washing bowl is filled with water at a suitable temperature; if tepid sponging is ordered, the water should be between 27°C and 32°C (80° to 90°F). Some patients will find a hot sponge, 43°C (110°F), more soothing; few patients, except perhaps in tropical countries, will appreciate cold sponging. The temperature of the water is not materially important; as already stated, the cooling of the body surface is brought about by evaporation.

The patient's face is first washed and dried; most people dislike having the face left wet, but the patient may find it comforting to have a cold compress on his forehead. The body is sponged in sections, beginning with one arm and using long sweeping strokes with the wet sponge. Spare sponges should be ready in the bowl of water, each sponge is used for two strokes only, using first one side then turning the sponge and using the other side; then it is put back in the water and a fresh sponge taken out. The sponge should be wet enough to leave small beads of moisture on the skin, which should not be dried. The whole procedure should take 15 to 20 minutes. At the end of the treatment the temperature is taken; it will in most cases continue to fall during the next thirty minutes and should be taken again at the end of that time.

When the moisture on the skin has evaporated, the bath blankets and mackintosh are removed and the nightgown is replaced. The patient is left covered with a sheet and, if necessary, one light blanket. Many patients will like to have a drink at the end of the treatment. If a cold compress has been used it is removed, the face is dried and the hair brushed.

The lowest point to which the temperature falls after sponging should be charted.

30 FIRST AID AND TREATMENT IN EMERGENCIES

First-aid treatment is confined to the help which a non-medical person can give in cases of accident or emergency until a doctor arrives. In all cases of serious injury the immediate concern of the helper is to get a doctor to the patient or to get the patient to hospital as quickly as possible. In the meantime first aid must be directed at maintaining life, preventing unnecessary suffering and keeping the victim's condition from worsening.

The immediate threats to life which must be dealt with promptly are:

(1) Cessation of breathing, which will quickly be followed by death unless resuscitation is started without delay.

(2) Profuse bleeding, which must be arrested as quickly as possible. This, fortunately, is not usually a difficult matter when dealing with external bleeding.

(3) Unconsciousness from any cause. An unconscious patient may lose his life unnecessarily if his airway is blocked by false teeth, or any foreign material, or by his own tongue, if he is left lying on his back.

Shock

Every seriously injured person will develop a degree of circulatory failure commonly known as "shock". The effect of this is slowing of the circulation and lowering of the blood pressure, leading to the condition of hypoxia, *i.e.* diminished oxygen supply to the tissue cells. Lack of oxygen leads to cerebral damage, cardiac, respiratory and renal failure. Blood loss is an important factor in producing a state of hypoxia and it should be remembered that the bleeding may not be obvious, as for example, bleeding into the tissues around a major fracture, such as a fractured femur.

There is no effective first-aid treatment for shock. Furthermore the signs of this condition, such as pale, cold skin and rapid pulse, may not be observable until a late stage, particularly in a healthy young adult. The first-aider should bear in mind that movement of an injured person increases shock and that any obvious urgent condition such as bleeding or a blocked airway must be looked for and treated.

The medical treatment is directed at increasing the volume of the circulating blood as quickly as possible. The nurse should prepare for the intravenous administration of plasma or plasma substitutes and the collection of a sample of blood for grouping and cross matching. Morphine is likely to be needed and may be given intravenously, as it will not be well absorbed from the subcutaneous tissues.

RESUSCITATION

If a person has ceased to breathe it follows that he has ceased to supply his body cells with vital oxygen. Unless breathing can be re-established within three to four minutes his brain cells will not recover from this oxygen deprivation. If the heart has stopped beating, even if oxygen is supplied to his lungs it cannot reach the brain. Therefore if no heart beat can be detected, cardiac as well as respiratory resuscitation is essential.

Respiratory Resuscitation

Speed is essential if artificial respiration is to be effective. Whatever method is used, the patient must be placed in position as quickly as possible, tight clothing must be loosened round his neck and waist, and his throat must be cleared of fluid and debris by turning the head to one side and sweeping round the mouth with a finger.

(1) Mouth to Mouth Method

The operator stands or kneels at the side of the victim, who must be lying on his back. The operator takes the patient's head in both hands, with one hand over the forehead and front of the head, presses the head back and extends the neck. The other hand is placed under the lower jaw pressing it forwards and upwards (Fig. 30.1). He then takes a deep breath, makes a seal with his lips

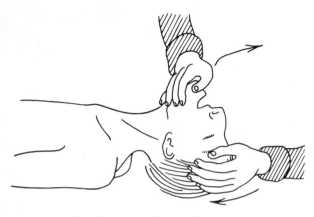

Fig. 30.1. MOUTH TO MOUTH RESUSCITATION.

The head is held in both hands and the casualty's jaw pushed upwards
and forwards.

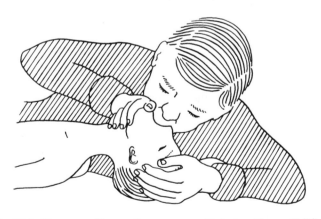

Fig. 30.2. MOUTH TO MOUTH RESUSCITATION (Infant or Young Child).

Seal your lips round the mouth and nose and blow gently until you see the
chest rise.

around the patient's mouth and closes the nostrils, either by resting his cheek against the nose or by pinching the nostrils, and blows into the mouth, watching for the patient's chest to rise. (Fig. 30.2). In the case of a child or a small adult the operator's lips must seal the nose as well as the mouth. He then removes his mouth, takes another deep breath and repeats the inflation. This should be done six times as quickly as possible. If the patient has not started to breathe spontaneously the procedure is continued at a rate of about 10 inflations per minute.

(2) Mouth to Nose Method

This method is preferred by some authorities as providing a better seal. It is also useful if the mouth cannot be opened, or if the casualty has no teeth when it may be difficult to obtain an effective seal. The procedure is the same as for mouth to mouth resuscitation except that the operator seals the patient's mouth with the thumb of the hand which holds up the chin; he then takes a deep breath, applies his mouth to the patient's face over the nose and blows into him.

Failure to inflate the lungs by either method usually means that the airway is obstructed at some point. Possibly the head is not

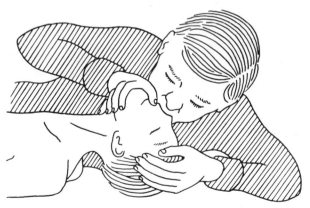

Fig. 30.3. MOUTH TO NOSE METHOD.

The lips are sealed on the casualty's face around the nose, and the thumb is placed on his lower lip to keep his mouth closed.

fully extended and therefore the airway behind the tongue is not open. The first thing to do is to check this and adjust the position if necessary. The operator should then look in the patient's mouth, for there may be some obvious blockage due to vomit or fluid which can be removed. It may be necessary to turn the patient on to his side and slap him smartly between the shoulder blades to dislodge foreign matter and empty out any fluid. A child may be held upside down and slapped between the shoulders.

Cardiac Resuscitation

If the heart has ceased to beat external cardiac resuscitation must be combined with respiratory resuscitation. Ideally, two operators should work together, one inflating the lungs and the other carrying out cardiac resuscitation.

Method

The operator places the ball of one hand over the lower half of the sternum. Having located this, he then puts his other hand on top of the first and gives six sharp presses over the area, depressing the chest about 3–4 cm. each time at a rate of about one per second. The second operator gives a mouth to mouth, or mouth to nose, inflation, then waits while the first operator repeats the series of presses over the sternum. While waiting to repeat the inflation this operator checks the pulse in the external carotid artery in the neck. As soon as the pulse returns the cardiac resuscitation is stopped, but mouth to mouth inflations must be continued until the patient is breathing naturally. If only one operator is available he should give alternately five mouth to mouth inflations followed by ten cardiac compressions until normal breathing and circulation are restored.

Practising these resuscitations is necessary if the first aider is to act promptly and efficiently when faced with a drowning accident or similar emergency. Members of a class may, quite understandably, not like the idea of blowing into each other's mouths. Various makes of teaching models are available, although most of them are rather expensive.

An inflating bellows, if available, can replace mouth to mouth breathing. One type of such apparatus is the "Cardiff" bellows.

This consists of a hand-operated bellows connected to an "ever-seal" mask. Compression of the fully extended bellows inflates the lungs, as is seen by the chest rising, and a valve which lifts when inflation ceases allows spontaneous expiration.

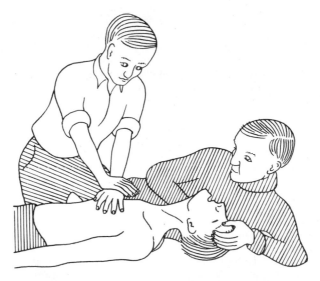

Fig. 30.4. EXTERNAL CARDIAC RESUSCITATION AND RESPIRATORY RESUSCITATION BEING UNDERTAKEN AT THE SAME TIME, TWO FIRST AIDERS WORKING ALTERNATELY.

Holger-Nielsen Method of Artificial Respiration

The Holger-Nielsen method was first introduced in Denmark. The essential movements in this method are back pressing and arm raising with the object of ventilating the lungs and stimulating cardiac action.

Immediate Action. Carry the patient quickly to a smooth flat place. Peel off tight or heavy clothing and loosen tight articles such as the collar and belt. In cases of drowning, clear the mouth of mud, sea-weed, etc., with the forefinger wrapped in a handkerchief.

Turn the Patient. If he is lying on his back, turn the patient into the prone position (*i.e.* face downwards).

Arrange Position of Patient. Arrange the patient's forehead on the support made by placing his hands one on top of the other. Make certain that his mouth and nose are completely unobstructed. If his mouth sinks towards the ground, raise his forehead an inch or so by placing the edge of a garment (*i.e.* a coat collar) under the hands. If necessary, turn the head slightly to one side.

Prepare for Artificial Respiration. (a) Slap the patient smartly once or twice between his shoulders. This usually causes the mouth to open, the tongue to fall forward, and, in drowning, to drive water out of the upper respiratory passages. If later it is found that the tongue is obstructing the passage of air, it must be drawn forward so that its tip protrudes slightly beyond the teeth.

(b) Place one knee 6–12 inches from the top of the patient's head, the inner side of the knee being in a straight line with the patient's cheek on the same side. Advance the other foot to the patient's elbow so that the heel is level with it and the toes point forward.

(c) Place both hands on the patient's back with the palms resting on the shoulder-blades, the thumbs on the spine, and the fingers pointing towards the feet (Fig. 30.5A).

Produce Expiration (pressure). Without bending the elbows and using no force whatever, rock the trunk gently forward on to the straight arms until they are vertical, thus exerting a smooth, gentle, evenly increasing pressure from above downwards on to the patient's back.

This movement should take 2 seconds, estimated by slowly counting—one, two, three (Fig. 30.5B).

Induce Inspiration (arm raising). (a) Counting four rock the trunk back allowing the hands to glide past the patient's shoulders until they can grasp his arms above the elbows.

(b) Using the straight arms, perform a steady, quick raising and pulling motion on the arms lasting 2 seconds, estimated by slowly counting—five, six, seven. Rock backwards a little, thus raising the patient's elbows to the level of his shoulders (Fig. 30.5C).

This action relieves the patient's chest of the weight of his trunk and lets the chest expand for a deep breath. The trunk itself must not be raised nor must the position of the hands be disturbed.

Continue Movements. On the count of eight, lower the arms to

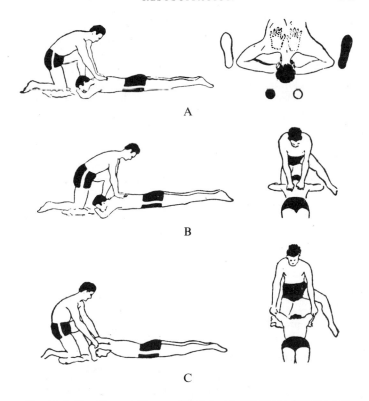

Fig. 30.5. THE HOLGER-NIELSEN METHOD OF ARTIFICIAL RESPIRATION.

the ground and move the hands to the initial expiration position in 1 second. Continue at the rate of 9 complete respirations per minute.

Signs of Recovery. When the patient shows signs of commencing recovery, continue artificial respiration until the improvement is established. Then continue with the arm-raising movement only, taking 2 seconds over each action of inspiration and expiration with no pause between them, *i.e.* 10 to 12 full respirations a minute.

Artificial respiration should be carried on until the patient breathes naturally or until a doctor has stated that the patient is dead. If the heart is still beating, there is hope that the patient may recover if artificial respiration is kept up.

At the same time other helpers should be directed to procure warm dry clothing and a warm bed prepared for the patient when he can be moved, or arrangements made to take him to hospital. Chest complications are very liable to follow.

Mechanical Respirators

If artificial aid is likely to be required over a long period, as in respiratory paralysis, some form of mechanical apparatus is used. The aim in all the various types of apparatus is to produce regular changes in pressure either on the lungs or inside the lungs in order that ventilation of the lungs may be maintained.

The three main types of apparatus are:

Negative-positive apparatus where negative pressure applied to the chest wall causes inspiration and expiration is produced by a slight degree of positive pressure.

Positive pressure apparatus where pressure is applied to the chest and inspiration is brought about by elastic recoil when the pressure is released.

Positive pressure through the airway, either by means of a face mask, an endotracheal tube or through a tracheostomy tube.

Negative-positive Pressure

The Drinker and the Both respirator and modifications of these consist of a steel cabinet in which the patient's body is totally enclosed except for his head. An airtight seal is provided by means of a sponge rubber collar which fits round the neck. When the patient needs attention while in the cabinet there are portholes through which the nurse can insert her arms, also one large enough for the insertion of a bedpan, and these are provided with a seal in the form of a rubber cuff. The cabinet can be tilted so that accumulation of secretions in the mouth and pharynx can be prevented by postural drainage. The pressure inside the cabinet is intermittently and rhythmically altered by an electrically driven pump, attached to the foot end of the cabinet by a length of unkinkable rubber hose pipe. The main disadvantage of this type of respirator is that nursing procedures are difficult to carry out. However, if the patient can continue breathing for short periods without the respirator, the bed on which he lies can be withdrawn from the cabinet and the necessary nursing attention can then be more efficiently given. If necessary the patient can be kept breathing by using anæsthetic apparatus for a short period. Provision must be made for the pump to be operated by hand in the event of a power failure. A handle is supplied which can be attached to a lever allowing manual operation to be brought into use in a few seconds should the motor fail. It is most important that nurses responsible for the care of a patient in a respirator should be familiar with the procedure of attaching the handle to the pump lever. Variations in the speed of the motor are possible, thus allowing for adjustment of the respiratory rate.

Positive Pressure to the Chest

An example of this type of apparatus is the Bragg-Paul respirator which consists essentially of an inflatable bag connected to a pump operated by an electric motor. The bag is fastened round the patient's chest and slightly inflated. The pressure in the bag is then alternately increased and decreased by the action of the pump. This apparatus is simple and can be worn when the patient is sitting up in a chair. Its chief use is to assist the patient who has some degree of movement in his respiratory muscles; it is not sufficient where paralysis is complete.

Positive Pressure through the Airway

The principle on which these resuscitators and respirators work is that the lungs are inflated by forcing air into the air passages.

The Oxford Resuscitator and various modifications of it are used for resuscitation over a short period. A regulating valve is attached to an oxygen cylinder connected to a rubber facepiece. The facepiece is fitted with a hand-controlled spring valve. When the spring is closed there is no escape of oxygen to the atmosphere and the gas is forced into the lungs. When the spring is released the flow of oxygen from the cylinder is cut off and the lungs are deflated by their own natural recoil.

The Beaver Type of Positive Pressure Apparatus. This is particularly useful when controlled respiration is required over a long period, as in the bulbospinal type of poliomyelitis, where respiratory paralysis is associated with paralysis of the pharynx and swallowing muscles.

A tracheostomy is performed and a cuffed rubber tube passed into the trachea. When the cuff is inflated the pharynx, nose and mouth are cut off from the rest of the respiratory tract and the secretions which the patient cannot swallow or expectorate can no longer enter the lungs. The tube is attached via an expiratory valve to a bellows type breathing bag which is alternately inflated and deflated by a small electrically driven motor. There is usually no need to supplement the oxygen in the normal room air in which the patient is being nursed, but if necessary oxygen can be added. Frequent suction is needed to keep the mouth and pharynx from "pooling" mucus and saliva. Feeding in these cases is carried out by means of an œsophageal tube passed through the nose into the stomach.

Carbon Monoxide Poisoning

The patient should be removed from the atmosphere contaminated by the gas into the fresh air. If he has ceased to breathe, artificial respiration should be started.

The best treatment is inhalation of oxygen or a mixture of oxygen and carbon dioxide, and therefore removal to hospital should be as prompt as possible.

Electric Shock

If the victim is still in contact with the electrical circuit and the current cannot be cut off, efforts must be made to pull him away from the live wire.

It is necessary to insulate the hands in some way, otherwise the current will pass from the victim to the would-be rescuer. First of all it should be remembered that water is a good conductor of electricity, therefore, if the ground is damp the rescuer should stand on a piece of dry wood, or on a thick woollen coat or rug. The victim should be grasped by the clothing and the rescuer's hands be protected with some insulating dry substance, such as any rubber material, folds of dry newspaper or clothing. If the patient cannot readily be reached, as, for example, if the accident occurred on an electric railway, he might be dragged from the live rail with the aid of wooden walking sticks with crooked handles. Umbrellas are dangerous on account of the metal spokes; all metals are good conductors of electricity.

If these efforts are successful, the first treatment to apply is artificial respiration. The burns sustained by the patient will have to be treated later.

CONTROL OF BLEEDING

Bleeding from a wound will in most cases stop spontaneously by the formation of a clot and shrinking of the ends of the cut vessels. A small blood loss is not serious; indeed it acts as a cleansing agent washing the wound. However, if large vessels are severed the victim may lose a great quantity of blood in a very short time and, as already stated, this blood loss will increase the circulatory failure which is a feature of serious injuries.

Most authorities now agree that a tourniquet has no place in first-aid treatment. It is not easy to apply it effectively and by obstructing the venous but not the arterial blood flow, it may well increase the bleeding. If the tourniquet succeeds in arresting the flow of blood it is likely to be damaging to the tissues and may even lead to ischæmic paralysis of muscles or gangrene of a limb. It is also generally accepted that pressure over the various arterial "pressure points", which has so long been a feature of first-aid teaching, is both difficult to achieve and time-wasting.

First aid in the treatment of profuse bleeding should aim at assisting the natural processes which enable the body to deal with blood loss.

Rest. The injured person should lie down with support and elevation of the wounded part. The blood flow to the area will then diminish and this will help closure of the ends of the cut vessels and the formation of a clot.

Pressure Directly on the Wound. This can be applied by holding a dressing firmly on the wound until such time as a bandage can be firmly applied. Pressure reduces the flow of blood and the dressing holds the shed blood and encourages clot formation.

In order to prevent infection of the wound a sterile first-aid dressing should be obtained if at all possible. If such is not available, then pressure may be applied with a large pad of any clean material to hand, such as a clean handkerchief or towel. If nothing at all is at hand and the bleeding is profuse from a large vessel, pressure can be exerted with the operator's bare hand.

In all cases where large quantities of blood have been lost it is essential to get the patient to a hospital where blood transfusion can be given.

In all cases too where the injury appears likely to have involved internal organs, or where internal bleeding is suspected, the patient must be taken to hospital without delay, but the first-aider should know what to do in certain special injuries and emergencies.

Bleeding from the Lungs

A crush injury or a stab wound in the chest is likely to injure the lungs and the patient, in addition to pain and difficulty in breathing, may cough up some blood. He will usually be most comfortable when propped up in a sitting or semi-sitting position. A puncture wound of the chest may be seen to suck air in every time the patient breathes. When air enters the chest cavity the lung on that side will collapse and, as the pressure increases, the action of the heart will be impeded and the opposite lung will be compressed. It is therefore necessary to prevent air entry as quickly as possible and this can be done by applying a large dressing and bandaging it very firmly round the chest.

Abdominal Wounds

In any injury which appears likely to have penetrated the abdominal cavity the patient must have immediate treatment in hospital. In the meantime no one must be allowed to give him anything whatever by the mouth.

Vomiting of blood is most often due to erosion of blood vessels in the stomach or duodenum by a peptic ulcer. The patient should be kept lying down while awaiting removal to hospital, and again nothing should be given by mouth. An estimate of the amount of blood vomited should be made and written down for the information of the doctor.

Ruptured Varicose Veins

Bleeding is profuse but easily arrested. The patient must lie down with the leg elevated. A firm dressing and bandage will usually control the bleeding at once. If, however, the first dressing becomes soaked and bleeding is obviously continuing, a second large pad or dressing should be applied over the first bandage and firmly secured.

Nose-bleeding (Epistaxis)

Nose bleeding from a blow on the nose usually stops spontaneously in a short time. Nose bleeding with no apparent cause is likely to be more troublesome. The patient should lie down with the head and shoulders elevated. Then direct him to pinch the nostrils firmly together while breathing through his mouth. If this is not effective or if the bleeding recurs, a doctor should see the patient.

UNCONSCIOUSNESS

"The first-aider who is faced with a patient who has been found, or has become unconscious, is not called upon to make a diagnosis. He must, however, make an immediate assessment of what has happened" (*First Aid in the Factory*, Lord Taylor).

It may be obvious that the unconscious person has sustained a severe head injury or that he has been overcome by coal gas poisoning, or there may be evidence that he has swallowed poison. In many instances, however, there may be no obvious indication of the cause and valuable time may be wasted in trying to decide this before attending to the patient.

It may be necessary to move the patient from danger, for example if he is in a gas-filled room; otherwise he should not be moved.

No unconscious person should be allowed to lie on his back; in this position his tongue will fall back, obstructing the airway, and saliva will collect in the throat. Not infrequently an unconscious patient may vomit and if he is on his back the vomit will almost certainly block the air passages and also be inhaled into the lungs. The first step then is to turn the patient over on to his face or into the semi-prone position so that his tongue falls forward and saliva and vomit can run out of his mouth. The first-aider should then see that the mouth is clear of any obstruction and hold the chin forward, so preventing the tongue from falling towards the back of the mouth.

If the patient is still unconscious when transported to hospital he must be kept in the prone or semi-prone position while being moved.

The first-aider should never attempt to rouse the patient or to put any fluid, such as brandy or water, into his mouth.

In all cases of unconsciousness medical aid must be obtained as soon as possible. The only exceptions to this rule are the simple fainting attack when the person recovers almost immediately, or an epileptic fit occurring in a known epileptic subject.

Some Common Causes of Unconsciousness

Head injuries. Head injuries may result from a blow on the head or from falling and striking the head, for example a person thrown from a bicycle in a skid or a collision. Motor cycle crashes at high speed have caused many fatal head injuries, hence the insistence on the safety precaution of wearing a "crash helmet". Any blow on the head which causes unconsciousness, even if only of a few moments' duration, should be regarded as a possibly serious injury and the patient must be seen by a doctor.

Cerebral damage from hæmorrhage or blood clot, "stroke". The patient is usually middle-aged or elderly. He may complain of feeling giddy and of loss of use of his arm and leg on one side of the body before he becomes unconscious. The immediate treatment is that described under "Unconsciousness". This patient quite obviously needs medical care and is usually admitted to hospital.

Epileptic fits. These fits can usually be easily recognized. The patient is unconscious and the fit proceeds through definite stages. It may be preceded by a warning, or aura, which is a sensory disturbance peculiar to the particular patient. The aura may be a vague feeling of discomfort, a flash of light before the eyes, or a sensation of dizziness. The aura may give the patient sufficient time to lie down before the fit begins.

The first stage of the fit observed by the onlooker is the tonic stage. The patient commonly gives a cry and falls to the ground unconscious. The muscles are rigid, respiratory movements cease, he becomes blue in the face and the eyes are turned upwards. This stage lasts about thirty seconds.

He then passes into the clonic or convulsive stage. The rigidity of the muscles passes off, to be succeeded by violent, jerky movements. The tongue is protruded and withdrawn, the patient foams at the mouth and may be incontinent. This stage lasts about sixty seconds.

Following the clonic stage, the patient passes into the stage of coma, often followed by sleep.

The only treatment necessary is to prevent any injury to the patient during the fit, and to remove him from any position of danger, for example near a fire. Tight collar-bands or waist-bands should be loosened. A soft gag may be put in the mouth in the clonic stage of the fit, but no force should be used. Epileptics have been known to have teeth, or even the jaw, broken by over-enthusiastic first-aiders during a fit.

FRACTURES AND JOINT INJURIES

Fractures

A fracture means a break in a bone. The two important classes of fracture are:
  (1) A simple or closed fracture, where there is no communica-
      tion between the site of the fracture and the external air.
  (2) A compound or open fracture, where there is a wound
      which forms a communication between the site of the frac-
      ture and the external air and therefore danger of infection.

Signs and Symptoms of a Fracture

  (1) Pain and tenderness over the site of the fracture.
  (2) Inability to move the arm or leg in the case of fracture of a
      limb.
  (3) Deformity: the limb is bent in a direction which would not
      be possible unless it were broken.
  (4) Bruising and swelling.

The history of the accident is often helpful; the patient may say that he felt the bone snap. Quite frequently the diagnosis can only be definitely made by an X-ray examination, and in all doubtful cases the first-aider should treat the injury as a fracture.

General Principles of Treatment

  (1) Avoid all unnecessary movement of the patient as this will
      cause pain and will increase the damage to the soft tissues

around the fracture, or may convert a closed fracture into an open one.

(2) Immobilize the part by the use of a splint before moving the patient. A variety of improvised splints may be used, *e.g.* suitable flat pieces of wood, umbrellas, pillows bandaged around the limb or the patient's own uninjured limb or the trunk.

(3) Cover any wound with the cleanest dressing available.

(4) Arrange for suitable safe transport of the patient.

Fractures of the Lower Extremity

Femur. Fractures of the neck of the femur commonly occur in elderly persons whose bones are brittle. The usual history is of a fall followed by pain in the hip and inability to stand. Fractures of the shaft of the femur are the result of considerable violence, for example in road accidents, and there is frequently considerable bleeding into the tissues of the thigh.

The limb should be splinted by applying a long wooden splint from the sole of the foot to just below the axilla and securing it by bandages round the chest, hips, upper part of thigh, above and below the knee and round the ankle and foot. An assistant should apply traction by pulling steadily on the foot, keeping it at a right angle to the leg, while the splint is applied. Another method is to bandage the injured limb firmly to the sound limb, with bandages round the hips, thighs, above and below the knee and around the ankle and foot. keeping the foot at a right angle to the leg.

Fractures of the tibia. The tibia has very little muscle covering and a fracture is usually obvious. The leg may be splinted by wooden splints, one on the outer side of the limb and a second shorter splint on the inner side. Another form of splinting uses a pillow which is wrapped around the leg and foot and firmly bandaged.

Fractures of the Upper Extremity

Humerus. A simple method of splinting a fractured humerus is to bandage the injured arm to the chest, or to pin the sleeve of the jacket to the chest and to support the forearm in a sling.

Radius and ulna. Fractures near the wrist joint (Colles's fractures) are usually the result of a fall on the outstretched hand.

Fractures of the shaft of these bones are commonly caused by direct violence. The forearm should be splinted from the elbow to the knuckles and a sling applied. Folded newspapers can be used to splint the forearm.

Clavicle (Collar bone). A fracture of this bone is often caused by a fall on the outstretched hand. There is not much risk of displacement of the broken ends of the bone if the arm is immobilized. The first-aid treatment is to put a pad in the axilla, bandage the upper arm to the chest and support the forearm in a St. John sling (Fig. 14.11).

Fracture of the Skull

The importance of these fractures is their liability to cause injury to the brain. Following a severe head injury the patient will be unconscious and may be bleeding from the ears and nose. There may be an escape of cerebrospinal fluid from the ear. First-aid treatment is that described for any unconscious patient. If clear fluid or blood is escaping from the ear a clean dressing may be applied. The patient must be taken to hospital as soon as possible.

Fracture of the Spine

If there is reason to suspect that a patient has a fractured spine, he should be kept lying still until sufficient help is at hand to lift him carefully on to a stretcher and convey him to hospital. It is important not to bend or twist the spinal column when moving the patient. The best position in which to transport him is lying on his back with small pillows or pads under the hollow of the neck, the small of the back and below the calves of the legs.

Fracture of the Pelvis

Fractures of the pelvis may injure the bladder, urethra or rectum. The patient should have a firm binder round the pelvis for support and should be lifted, without rolling, on to the stretcher.

Fracture of the Ribs

The special danger of a broken rib is that the ends of the bone may damage the lung. Following the injury the patient may complain of great pain on breathing and may cough up blood.

It is essential that medical aid should be sought early, as chest complications are apt to occur, especially in elderly patients.

The first-aid treatment consists of supporting the patient in the most comfortable position, usually sitting up.

Joint Injuries

Dislocations

A dislocation is a displacement of the joint surfaces of two or more bones and is accompanied by damage to the soft tissues around the joint.

Signs and Symptoms

(1) Deformity.
(2) Pain.
(3) Loss of movement.
(4) Swelling.

The shoulder joint is fairly readily dislocated; fingers, the elbow joint, knee joint and jaw may also be dislocated comparatively easily, but considerable violence is needed to dislocate the hip joint.

The first-aid treatment consists of supporting the part with a sling or bandages. A dislocation is most easily reduced immediately after the injury, therefore no time should be lost in obtaining medical aid.

Sprains

A sprain is an injury to the soft tissues of a joint involving the muscles and ligaments. The usual situations are the ankle, wrist and thumb.

Signs and Symptoms

(1) Pain.
(2) Swelling.
(3) Discoloration.

Treatment

The possibility of a dislocation or a fracture should be considered and the patient urged to get medical attention. In the meantime he should not use the limb and some support may be

given by the application of a firm bandage. Elevation of the part
and cold applications may help to prevent swelling.

BURNS AND SCALDS

A burn is an injury produced by dry heat, and a scald by moist
heat. From the point of view of first aid the immediate results of
the injury and the treatment are the same. Burns are likely to en-
danger life immediately as a result of loss of plasma from the
burnt area and depletion of the volume of circulating blood. It
should be understood that the patient's life is in danger from an
extensive burn, even if it be entirely superficial; if one quarter of
the total skin surface is involved the injury is extremely serious.

Medical aid should be obtained as speedily as possible. Full
treatment of the burnt area will be carried out only in hospital,
but morphine may be required immediately for the relief of pain.
The patient should be moved as little as possible and gentle
handling is essential. A burnt patient may complain of thirst and
small amounts of water may be given to relieve this. It is better to
give small quantities frequently rather than to encourage the
patient to drink large amounts as vomiting is not unusual.

The burnt area, if exposed, should be covered with the cleanest
dressing to hand, if sterile dressings are not available clean towels
or sheets may be used as substitutes. The surface which has been
folded in, and therefore protected from dust should be placed
next to the burnt skin. Blankets and rugs should not be allowed
to come in contact with an exposed burnt area as they are poten-
tial sources of heavy bacterial contamination. If the injured area
is covered by clothing this is best left undisturbed.

When the patient is admitted to hospital his immediate needs
for fluid replacement are assessed. In all serious cases transfusion
is started at once, usually with plasma or plasma substitutes.
Blood may also be needed as, particularly in deep burns, there is
considerable destruction of red blood cells.

Where burns are likely to be common accidental injuries, as for
instance in certain industries, the use of a water-soluble cream
containing penicillin or sulphonamide and 1 per cent. cetrimide
is one of the dressings recommended for use in first aid. Any first-
aid dressing should be carried out with all the aseptic precautions
that the circumstances permit. The dresser should wash her hands

and dry them on a clean towel before handling any dressing material and an improvised mask, *e.g.* a clean pocket handkerchief, should be worn.

Scalds of the Throat and Mouth

Such accidents may occur in young children, who may suck the spout of a teapot or boiling kettle.

Medical aid should be obtained at once; swelling of the upper air passages may cause obstruction of the air way and tracheostomy may be necessary. The child should be put to bed and kept warm.

Chemical Burns

The chemical should be thoroughly washed off with warm water. If the nature of the substance is known, a neutralizing agent may be used, *e.g.* a corrosive acid such as nitric acid should be washed off with a solution of sodium bicarbonate or lime water. Strong lysol or carbolic acid splashed on the skin is best removed with surgical spirit or methylated spirit. Caustic soda burns may be treated with a weak acid such as vinegar.

Chemical Burns of the Eye. The eye should be opened (an assistant may be needed to do this) and then thoroughly washed out with clean water for at least fifteen minutes. The eye is then covered with a pad and bandage. Medical treatment is essential and urgent in order to prevent permanent damage.

POISONING

Poisoning by accident is a not uncommon emergency; children may swallow fluids or tablets left within their reach, adults may drink a supposed dose of medicine from an unlabelled bottle or may fail to read the label and swallow a dose of disinfectant or cleaning fluid. Deliberate taking of poison is usually with suicidal intent but may be the act of a hysterical person who wants to attract sympathy. Deliberate administration of a poison is of course done with the object of killing, or at least seriously harming, the victim.

The immediate course of action to be taken by the first-aider is to send urgently for medical aid and to try to find the nature of the

EXAMPLES OF TYPES OF POISONS, SYMPTOMS PRODUCED AND APPROPRIATE FIRST-AID TREATMENT

Poison	Signs and Symptoms	Treatment
1. *Corrosive poisons,* e.g. phenol or Lysol.	Burns on lips and mouth. Intense pain from mouth to stomach. Vomiting. Marked shock. Thirst.	Immediate treatment, dilute the poison by giving tap water or milk if the patient can swallow. If the poison is a coal tar disinfectant, a stomach wash-out, using 1 per cent. solution of magnesium sulphate (Epsom salts), should be prepared; 2 fl. ozs. of liquid paraffin may be put down the tube after the wash-out.
2. *Irritant poisons,* e.g. mercury preparations, arsenic.	Pain in abdomen. Vomiting; the vomit may contain blood and mucus. Diarrhœa. Collapse.	Give an emetic, prepare for stomach wash-out. Treat collapse by warmth and hot applications to abdomen. Following the emetic or wash-out a demulcent mixture of milk and egg may be given.
3. *Poisons acting on the nervous system:* Hypnotic and narcotic poisons, e.g. morphine, barbiturates.	Drowsiness, coma, slow respirations.	If the poison has been swallowed, give an emetic. Prepare for stomach wash-out. Stimulate patient by giving strong coffee, inhalation of smelling salts or ammonia. Artificial respiration if necessary. The specific antidote to opium or morphine is nalorphine which combats respiratory failure. Drugs used to combat the effect of barbiturates include nikethamide, Methedrine and bemegride.
Convulsant poisons, e.g. strychnine	Restlessness, delirium, convulsions.	Emetic and stomach wash-out, if seen early. If patient is having convulsions, keep as quiet as possible. Drugs used to combat the convulsive poisons include anaesthetics such as thiopentone sodium and muscle relaxants e.g. tubocurarine, Scoline.

poison so that an appropriate antidote can be obtained and to
dilute the poison (if swallowed) as rapidly as possible. The nearest
diluent to hand is usually water and the victim should drink four
or five tumblerfuls of water at once. If it is readily available,
milk is a good diluent and demulcent fluid. Unless there is evidence of a corrosive poison (burning of the mouth and lips) the
first-aider should try to induce vomiting. This may be effected by
putting the fingers down the victim's throat or giving an emetic
such as salt, two tablespoonfuls, or one teaspoonful of mustard, in
a glass of warm water.

Examples of some common types of poisons, symptoms and
treatment are given in the table on page 359.

INDEX

THIS BOOK HAS BEEN SET IN MONOPHOTO TIMES NEW ROMAN AND MADE AND PRINTED BY OFFSET IN GREAT BRITAIN BY WILLIAM CLOWES AND SONS, LIMITED, LONDON AND BECCLES, FOR BAILLIÈRE, TINDALL AND COX, LIMITED